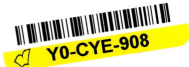
FEARLESS SPIRIT
JOYOUS
HEART

BRING YOUR SOUL TO LIFE

LEE PARORE

> ❝ *What lies behind us and what lies before us are tiny matters compared to what lies within us* ❞
>
> **OLIVER WENDELL HOLMES**

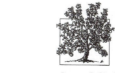

www.applepublishing.com

Copyright © 2004 by Lee Parore and Apple Publishing Co. Ltd.
Layout and Cover Art by Thomas Conley Design

Apple Publishing Company reserves all rights to this edition. No part of this work may be repro-
duced or transmitted in any form or by any means, electronic or mechanical, including photo-
copying and recording, or by any information storage or retrieval system, except those wishing
to quote brief passages in connection with a review.

Printed in Canada

National Library of Canada Cataloguing in Publication Data

Parore, Lee, 1962-
  Fearless spirit, joyous heart : bring your soul to life! / Lee Parore.

  ISBN 1-896817-44-0

  1. Self-actualization (Psychology) 2. New Age movement. I. Title.
BF637.S4P37 2003   158   C2003-910337-4

Apple Publishing Company Ltd.
220 East 59th Avenue
Vancouver, British Columbia
Canada V5X 1X9 Tel. (604) 214-6688 Fax. (604) 214-3566

E-mail: books@applepublishing.com   Website: www.applepublishing.com

10   9   8   7   6   5   4   3   2   1

Dedicated to three generations of women...

My Mother, Joy
My Partner, Emma
My Daughter, Jasmin

Thank you for your support, inspiration
and unconditional love.

CONTENTS

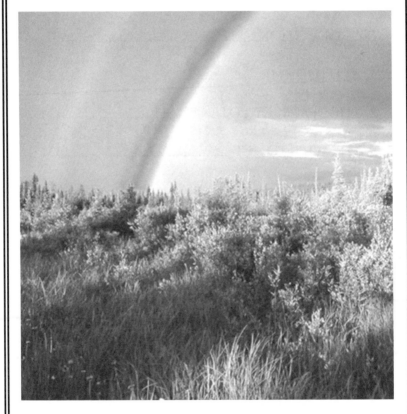

Life is the interplay of forces. By living in accordance with principles of wholeness we can embrace our full potential.

INTRODUCTION

Fearless Spirit - Joyous Heart is a stand for the sacred. To embrace the universal wisdom of consciousness that resides within us. *Our Soul.* The part of us linked energetically, with all sentient beings. Our Soul is our *individual energy,* of which our personality is a part. By merging our souls intuitive guidance with our personalities need to express creatively its intention and desire, we become a *whole being.* We bring balance to our energy. The road to our Soul is through our Heart. Here we find our Spirit

In essence life is what we make it. The choices we decide and the efforts we initiate determine the life we experience. More important though is the person we become during the course of our lifetime. There are infinite possibilities, but ultimately only two paths of journey.

We can either run from all that we are or we can delve into the wholeness of all that we are. The choice is ours - to evolve towards fulfilling our full potential.

Our true nature is creative. Just as nature's cycle is one of birth and death, the creation and recycling of all things is our natural way. The capacity to adapt intuitively and change with change as life evolves around us, and still maintain the integrity of our character. This journey requires us to bare our soul, the essence of who we are, honestly and totally. The ultimate creativity is to live mortality.

Life owes us nothing. It is up to us to pay our dues and sow the seeds we wish to reap. What's inside ignites us, our determination and motivation is the key to our success. Our first admission is to realize that we must take responsibility for our own life.

Resonate with what makes our soul sing, follow our hearts path and allow our true self to shine. Nothing meaningful in life manifests until we face and know the full power of our whole self. This requires the willingness to open our mind to all possibilities, and to self-initiate the willpower to focus on creating what we want from life.

Belief and courage are keys. The belief in our self and the courage to persevere in the face of adversity strengthens our creative spirit for life. The courage to face our fears and the belief that life's rewards are based upon the intent of our actions opens our heart, which brings our soul to life. Anything less is too weak to make us strong enough to undergo the metamorphosis that leads to living an authentic, soulful life. Whereby we open the inlet to live artfully in life's constant stream of possibilities.

Actions speak the truth. Our code of conduct determines the relationships we create with our self and others. The capacity to be firm in our actions, but not weak marks the difference. Life tests us at our most crucial times. It is our response, how we manage our self, that forms the person we are today. When we base integrity as the mainstay of our behavior, we align our actions to live to life's highest truths in the eternal moment of here and now.

Our heart is our true home. Here we align our personalities ego with the wisdom of our soul's essence. We bring meaning and pleasure into our life. The jewels of joy emanate from an open heart, the true inlet from which we merge intellect with love. Love is life's highest energy, from which we unconditionally serve our own growth and rejoice in the creative growth of others. We must endeavor to remain fearless in our approach and joyous in our participation. Aim to evolve towards the best we can be.

By bringing our soul to life we merge with life's infinite web of creation. Our ability to embrace our wholeness is what allows us to dance our song and enjoy the journey.

A human being is a part of a whole called by us "universe", a part limited in time and space. We experience our self, our thoughts and feelings as something separated from the rest.... a kind of optical delusion of consciousness. This delusion is a kind of prison for us, restricting us to our personal desires and to affection for a few persons nearest to us. Our task must be to free ourselves of this prison by widening our circle of compassion to embrace all living creatures and the whole of nature in its beauty.

ALBERT EINSTEIN

KEYS TO THE SOUL

1. *Take full responsibility for this Life*

2. *Open our creative mind to possibilities*

3. *Become Conscious of our thoughts and actions*

4. *Center our Energy - Expand our awareness*

5. *Integrate Personality and Soul - Wholeness*

6. *Have Faith and Courage*

7. *Open our Heart - Raise our level of consciousness*

8. *Let Love with Peace - Be the energy that guides us*

9. *Embrace all as Family*

CHAPTER 1

IT'S ABOUT ATTITUDE

 To refuse to be cast down,
that is the lesson.

Walk on and see a new view.

Walk on and see the birds fly.

Walk on and leave behind all
things that would dam up
the inlet of experience.

BRUCE LEE

Life is about waking up with a smile on our face, feeling good about who we are and what we do. It's an outward journey reflecting an inward journey that emanates from our attitude towards life. How we handle the contrasting aspects of our inner nature determines *the power we harness* to create our life. Like the two faces of a coin, Fearless Spirit, Joyous Heart is "an attitude" that unites the essence, *the soul* of who we are into a state of wholeness. To cultivate the desire to make the most of our self as we endeavor to experience life fully.

Fearless Spirit is the *peaceful warrior* in us all, skilled in the art of *self-control* and total body-mind *advancement*. Our spirit provides us with the will to initiate action with the utmost sincerity. With spirit we're able to stand up for our self and for the rights of others. We possess the boldness to speak for the good of the higher cause, for family, planet earth and for life itself. The fearless warrior has honor, self-knowledge and is committed to growth with integrity.

Joyous Heart is the *lover* in us all, skilled in the art of *giving* and *receiving*. Our heart keeps us in touch with our deepest feelings and personal truths. From our heart comes inner peace with a strong sense of self-worth. We possess the sensitivity to respond with compassion and the courage to act intuitively without discrimination. The joyous lover is considerate towards all life, with a heart of gold and love for all beings.

Fearless Spirit and Joyous Heart are mutually dependent attitudes for a life of honest expression. Like the polarities, positive and negative, yin and yang, masculine and feminine, without which there would be no atomic matter, no existence, no relationships and certainly no *inner force* to urge us to evolve. The *unity of diversities* provides the catalyst for our *creative growth*. In time our attitude becomes our way, forming the foundation for

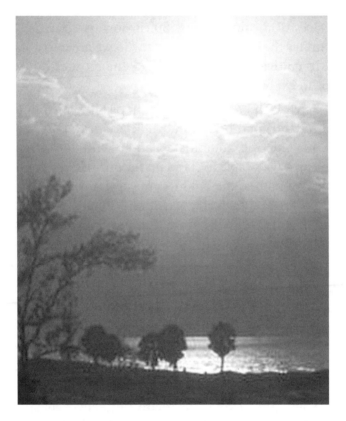

Each day life invites us to shine. Express with attitude, this is to be our own experience.

the life we experience. Without a fearless spirit how can we become all we wish to be? Without a joyous heart, what's the point? Life should be fun and fulfilling. Fearless Spirit, Joyous Heart gives us a sense of belonging to a greater universal entity with an awareness of our *individual power* and place in *the web of life.*

Our journey from mother's womb to death's tomb is an evolutionary process towards our consummate best. What drives and sustains us to become our best is our attitude. Without motivation and determination we lack the spirited energy necessary to open our heart and participate in life. Our attitude is the *fuel that ignites our inner strength,* the source of our inspiration to be adaptive with life. In essence, our attitude becomes the *song of our soul* as it beats forth the rhythm of *how we dance* with life. Being soulful ensures our actions stay aligned towards the benefit of our self and for the good of humankind.

Fearless Spirit and Joyous Heart are the *seeds of power* to our potential. Each of us are born with genetic strengths, gifts and talents, it's what we do with them that determines our future. Take responsibility for this life, embrace our creativity and walk forever with the *heart of a joyous lover* and the *spirit of a fearless warrior.* The *choice is ours.*

ENERGY WAITING TO HAPPEN

Albert Einstein's famous formula $E=MC^2$ showed us matter and energy are interchangeable. That matter is a manifestation of energy. In layman's terms, we're a *mass of energy waiting to happen.* Energy in the form of thoughts and feelings command our will, thus determining our actions. Everything we do involves energy, the way we think and feel, breathe and move all influence the sum flow of energy throughout our body and therefore the form we take. It is the choices we make, and what we do with our energy that shapes us. We are what we think and feel, a *manifestation of our consciousness.* Einstein showed that the *energy is inside the mass;* therefore the power to become all that we can be is within us.

Energy is the currency of life. Our *thoughts* transmit invisible energy we call attitude at the speed of light. This influences what doors open for us, and the course our life takes. We can choose to live with an *ego consciousness* whereby our thinking diminishes who we are and limits our opportunities. Or we can choose to live with a *universal consciousness* whereby our thinking expands upon who we are and welcomes limitless growth. Energy works best for us when it comes from the belief that all things are interdependent, with our soul and personality merged. Ultimately, the level of our consciousness is determined by our attitude. Fearless Spirit, Joyous Heart is about cultivating the will to master our mind. Being *the creator of our life,* within life's web.

Our body emits a vibrating field of energy that changes moment to moment in response to events taking place. There are two directions in which this *resonant field of energy* can move, *towards expansion* or *towards contraction.* Encoded within us since birth is the basic instinct to grow, to expand our identity. The basic impulse of life is to reach outward. Only through the *expansion of our inner self* can we reciprocate a positive flow-back of energy from which to manifest the life of our dreams. When we take action solely for our own benefit, we block our energy flow. We diminish our capacity to interact creatively in life. In time it collapses inward with nowhere to go. Selfish awareness with attention to ones own ego at the expense of others eventually brings isolation and inevitable pain. Energy expressed joyfully and given willingly for the good of all, behaves like the infinite universe, circulating and recycling energy abundantly. Our energy flows best when our actions are aligned with the *responsibility for all life.*

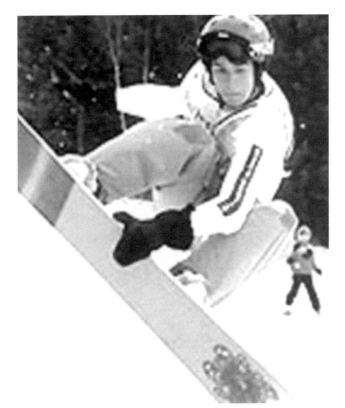

The body operates a trinity of power. The brain is home to our intellectual and visionary powers. The heart is home to our feelings from where we resonate with what feels right. The belly is the gravitational center of our body, home of our physical power. What we do with our power determines who we become.

We are potential energy, what we think, feel and allow our self to be. What matters is what we do and how we act. People instinctively sense our *personal energy*, which either *attracts or repels* whatever we want in life. Energy created by our thoughts and feelings spreads throughout our body, out into the space around us projecting a magnetic force that attracts our desires or the objects of our expectations. Whatever we direct our energy towards creates our perception, which becomes our reality. The stronger our will towards our desire, the greater is our flow of energy towards its manifestation. Whatever energy we put out flows back to us reinforced by the truth of our actions. To attract the things that bring us joy we must *be crystal clear* in choosing our thoughts and responses to life's experiences, for they determine our future.

RESONATE WITH LIFE

Energy cannot be created or destroyed. It can only be transformed from one state to another. The energetic effect of our attitude is the same. The form energy takes depends upon its *vibrational frequency*, which is directly influenced by the way we think, feel and behave. When we lose the ability to *joyfully express our self* we diminish our power to truly *resonate with life*. When we are enthused about what we are currently doing, we increase our power to resonate with life. It is our intent and *emotional charge* for things that illuminates our life.

Every body is a mass of energy urged on by an inner force, our attitude. Remember how much lighter we feel, and freer we think when we dance, and how the entire world looks better when we're in love. Changing the way we feel and think internally changes the world we experience externally. As the scientist Nikola

Tesla stated over 100 years ago, *"mass of a higher velocity is the key"*. By shifting our attitude towards principles based upon being more positive and constructive, we lift our energy and *raise our level of consciousness* to a more creative realm. The very *spirit of our being resonates a vibration* that we sense deep in the core of our body. The urge to become more conscious of our self, the way we interact in the world and its repercussions. The vibes of a resonating inner attitude reflects an aura of warm-hearted vitality, and inner poise.

We operate a trinity of power, a system of intelligence consisting of *mind, body* and *emotions*. The brain is our *thinking center*. It governs our state of consciousness, and is the mind's eye from which we view life. It is the conductor for hormonal drive and the *central command center* of the body-mind nervous system. The heart is our *feeling center* that prevents us from becoming an android. It is our internal metronome from which we *resonate with what feels right* for us in life. It produces the strongest electrical and magnetic activity of any tissue in our body and is the power pump that keeps us alive. The belly is our *action center*. It is home to our center of gravity, and the *vortex of our energy* from which we plug into life. Each center influences and is dependent upon the others for optimal health and peak performance. Synchronizing these energy reservoirs magnifies our innate power to fulfill the wholeness of our potential.

Life demands we have the brains, the heart and the guts to sustain our authenticity, the essence of who we are. Mind and body co-exist as one. Ultimately our direction in life is determined by our capacity to think, feel and take action cohesively. One without the other is incomplete. Integrating our physical, mental and emotional unifies intellect and instinct enhancing our spontaneity to *feel from our heart*, to *use our head wisely* and *have the guts* to energetically live our dreams.

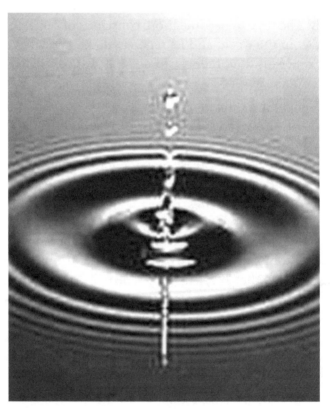

*Like a pebble dropped into water our
thoughts radiate to the world that which we are. By
shifting our attitude we transform our life.*

The way we resonate with life is *our conscious choice.* Through life experience we gain insights as to whether we're truly allowing our self to shine. If we need to *shift our attitude to transform our life,* then do so. Change is about trading the things that hold us back in life for the things that *make our soul sing.* Our ideas and beliefs form the structure of our experience. Chance favors those who positively create their own future.

SPIRIT OF SELF-INQUIRY

Those who seek the answers to life outside of themselves, spend a lifetime looking. The inlet to life's power resides in our ability to *know our self* and to be *true to our self.* Only from the perspective of *self-awareness* can we create the life we aim to experience. It is our mind that lay's the foundation to win this internal battle, to *trust our self.* To know our self we must be fully conscious of our thoughts, emotions and actions. Self-inquiry is the pathway to *self-knowledge,* to living a *life of truth* through self-awareness. We empower our self with the *authentic attitude* that emanates our intent to *honor all that we are.*

Self-inquiry is about questioning our inner chatter and examining our external actions. Everything we do is an *opportunity to know* more deeply who we are and how we operate, to query our motives. When there is discord within we manifest disharmony in our outer lives. When we can identify the disparity between our inner and outer worlds we can rid ourselves of destructive habits. We can then direct our will to integrate happiness, fulfillment, inner peace, and contentment to become our unshakeable shadow.

Life is a *self-fulfilling prophecy.* It is up to us to create the life we wish to live. Self-inquiry is the first step in transforming the way we think and feel. To integrate the creativity of our personal-

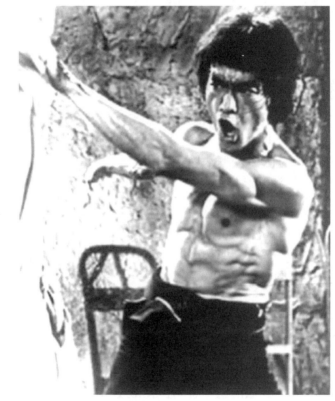

Martial arts phenomena Bruce Lee was all about living with an expressive creative attitude, the essence of Fearless Spirit, Joyous Heart.

ity with the truths we discover about our self and life. Harmonizing our inner world ensures clarity of mind and razor sharp focus with a healthier self-image, the hallmarks for successful behavior. It builds within us the *fearless character* and *joyous disposition* capable of handling failure whilst continuing with nondestructive ruthlessness towards our goals. Staying *true to our self* builds self-confidence and inner resolve. This is the difference between seeking that which makes us feel good about our self and that which enables us to become more of our self.

Our opportunities reside within us. The car we drive, the clothes we wear, the house we live in, are all external. They're symbols of the personal images we place before the world. They may make us feel good, but aren't necessarily *what makes us great.* They don't guarantee happiness, health or wealth. It's what's inside us that counts, the heart and the spirit we have for life. At the center of our life is the interconnectedness of our thinking, feeling and doing, our way of being human. When the going gets tough our inner world holds the key to our responses. The way we *manage our experiences* ultimately determines how we grow and develop as a person.

Those wanting to journey within to understand the deeper mechanisms of self should be prepared to discover good and bad, the multitudes of human nature. The realization that our mind is at the root of our being, and its capacity to overcome obstacles at times wavers, is key. The spirit of self-inquiry allows us to pierce the façade our mind's ego has built around us, that *life is what we've made it.* Our perception has become our reality, its meaning gives birth to our actions. Our limits in life are our beliefs, which are based upon our interpretation of things. Self-inquiry awakens *self-awareness,* the wellspring from which authentic self-expression emanates with the capacity to live in harmony with our self. Being true to others becomes an act, whereas *being true to our self is reality.*

WE REAP WHAT WE SOW

There is an ancient story about a man walking through a mountainous country with rocky cliffs all around him. As he shouts aloud, the mountains send his words back to him. This phenomena is known as, the *law of echo reflection*. The sound of his voice strikes the cliff walls and bounces back, just as a ball bounces when it hits the ground. The same patterns are repeated in life, we emit a ceaseless flow of waves, beneficial or noxious through our thoughts, feelings and behavior. These waves journey through space until they come against the outer limits and bounce back to strike the sender in the form of rewards or punishment. It's like there's a certain number of laws within and around us that govern us. Prosperity and adversity come in their own time through the effects of our actions. In essence, *tomorrow is earned today*. The secret is to *sow the seeds we want*.

We *receive* from the world what we *give* to the world. This is life's golden law, to *give unconditionally*, and to *receive unconditionally*. This is ecology, the natural distribution of life's energy, to ensure sooner or later we *accept responsibility* for our attitude. Our every thought, feeling and action is motivated by an *intention* and *desire*, which becomes a cause that exits as one with an effect. Every cause that hasn't yet manifest an effect is an event that has not yet come to completion in our life. Our soul is that part of us that keeps record of all we do, it doesn't judge. It is our teacher to living life from the perspective of a higher consciousness. At the end of the day our ego's personality answers to our soul. *Everything goes full circle*, back to us! The deeper we *resonate from our core* the more of our soul we bring to life.

Life is energy. Our thoughts create our attitude, which ultimately determines our actions and our life direction. Everything in life we earn, the result of our efforts or as the eastern sages remind us *we reap what we sow*. We all have problems that we have to confront and solve in life. What makes the difference is what we do with them. As the master said to the disciple, "good luck follows sincere effort". When our heart and spirit aren't immersed in what we do, our actions become weak. We lack depth and substance. When our heart and spirit are deeply involved there is depth and joy in everything we do. No matter what life brings, we have the power to *discipline our attitude* and way of life. The way we think and behave during both fortunate and turbulent times determines our life experience. Endeavour to refrain from negative actions, engage in virtuous actions and help others.

If we are to be our *own master of fate*, we must confront our crosses of destiny. Moments when we must choose which way to go, the known or the unknown, to travel the path of lightness or darkness. We have the choice to let ourselves slide into a life of sloth and pleasure to avoid difficulties, to neglect work and responsibility. But there is no escape until we have solved the problems the world has set before us to teach us the lessons we need to learn. To endeavor to understand what they mean and to do whatever has to be done to overcome them. Learn to *solve problems* by means of wisdom, love and purity. In life the universe helps those whom help themselves, those whom accept authentic responsibility for their destiny. Divine justice is based on *living in accordance with love*, only then will we become that which we feel and think we deserve.

SOUL KEYS

*We are a mass of energy waiting to
happen - Our attitude is what ignites us
It determines the person we become*

*We are what we think and feel, a
manifestation of our consciousness -
take action towards being soulful*

*Resonate with Life -
What makes the soul sing?*

*Self-inquiry brings the self-knowledge and
awareness that leads to a life of truth -
to live with soul*

We reap what we sow - It is our choice

CHAPTER 2

THE REALM OF POTENTIALITY

> *We are what we think. All that we are arises with our thoughts, and with our thoughts we make our world.*
>
> **THE BUDDHA**

THE POWER OF VISION

We choose what we create. The thoughts we entertain project an image onto the inner screen of our mind. The more focused our thoughts, the clearer our brain conceptualizes it as reality. In essence, life is the realm of possibility, and *we are pure potentiality*, whereby everything and anything is possible. It is from our mind's eye that we choose our thoughts and create an artists impression to manifest what we want in life. The key in this process is to meditate upon our desire, and let our creativity unfold.

Clear vision precedes great accomplishments. We architecturally design our future through our minds vision. Our thoughts initiate laser-like missiles that *sight our target* and launch towards actual manifestation. The reality of our experience depends upon the nature of our thoughts. Negative thoughts manifest experiences of suffering. Positive thoughts manifest experiences of joy. To be mindful of the thoughts we entertain is our responsibility. To be careful what we wish for is our prime consideration. Target and *tune to the positive*, the higher realms of our consciousness. This inspires us to manifest more creative designs in our mind.

Our visions form the *blueprint* of our reality. The images we picture in our mind most frequently are stored as reality by our central nervous system. Our body then responds to these images as beliefs. These form the perspective from which we view the world and live our life. In essence, what we conceive, we can achieve. To align our life with what we truly want to experience, we must repeatedly visualize what we intend to manifest. The key in this process is to *feel the essence* of what we want as an *impulse in our heart*. The deeper we resonate our intention, the stronger our belief fulfills our vision. When every cell in our body feels the

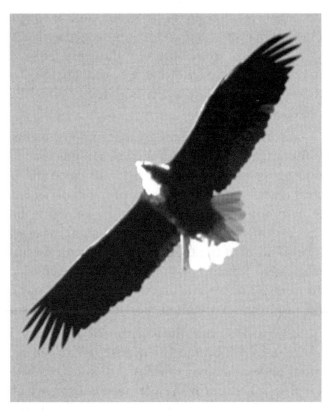

*Like the eagle, harness the minds eye and
conceptualise the destiny of choice.*

vision of our mind, we are able to summon and direct all our energy towards our objectives becoming reality.

Our life is constructed from images held within our mind. To become all we can be and journey where we wish to travel, we must *live more consciously*. By cultivating more awareness of the thoughts and images we entertain we can alter our focus to create a *statement of purpose* for our life. Remember, our ideas and visions precede the course our life takes. We get from life what we expect, what we program into our own mind. By holding specific images with heart-felt desire we build the bridge that brings our visions into realization. Only that which takes root in our mind can become factual reality in our life. Only then can we naturally gravitate towards creating an *original life.*

What we focus on grows within. Our body as well as our head forms the field from which we experience everything in life. The vehicle to bring our visions to life is our body, where we grow into an understanding of how to deliver our goals. When we hold firm to our vision, our body in time senses the culmination of our rational mind and our feeling heart. We then experience the surge of energy in the core of our body urging us to take action in accordance with what we see. This creates the power to *take ownership of our life* and to single-mindedly strive towards accomplishing our goals. What comes to us is in the end, is only that which we've been accepting in consciousness.

THE MIND'S EYE

Our mind contains the power to create our destiny of choice. Whatever we *visualize* or *imagine* we invite into our life. The limit to what we can manifest is our imagination. The key question requiring a crystal clear answer is *what do we want?* Our mind works like a boomerang with our pictured thoughts returning to us in the form of physical reality. When we view our mind as being the creative force, we become aware that life is full of limitless opportunities. Our mind's eye is the *realm of possibility*, the creative haven to conjure up ideas that change and improve our world.

Our *creative mind* is our *magic wand*. Kids naturally access the mind's eye as they indulge in the playful art of daydreaming. Many adults forget the simple gift of spending a moment in time to imagine and create a *life of joy*. We are often swept up in the hustle and bustle of modern day living, obsessed with keeping up with the Joneses. The first person we need to take care of and make happy is our self. This is only possible when we accept responsibility for our own life unfolding. That which brings us joy is often different to that which brings someone else joy. Societal beliefs are set before us as boundaries preventing us from straying too far from the norm. Notice how each new generation will *challenge the limits* to see new ways of living life. Our future happiness is created through the power of our imagination, revealing to us what is possible. Each of us must take fearless action with a joyous disposition towards manifesting our own foreseen reality. We can become our future, when we continue to imagine our self, and our surrounding set of circumstances living the life of our dreams in full color.

Our mind's eye gifts us a *language* inexpressible in words, beyond the scope of our brain's intellect. It connects us to a bigger picture of the possibilities within us, a power that we're only beginning to tap into. Possessing the *power of vision* gets us started on the road to experiencing everything and manifesting anything. The more we accept we create our own reality through our mind's eye, the more consciously we tune to the flow of thoughts and images we see before us, to create and manifest actual reality.

To enter the mind's eye, *experience silence.* The kid who stares up into the sky daydreaming welcomes flashes of intuitive insights. Einstein was often quoted as saying; "I arrived at none of my major theories through rational thought". Indulging our self in the world of creative imagination enables us to learn and create concepts beyond analysis and reasoning alone. It allows our *mind to wonder,* as children do, and gives us the opportunity to reply with the deepest expression of our being. It gives us access to an *in between place* that brings totality, a balance between fantasy and reality.

To deepen the experience of the mind's eye, *spend time alone.* Relax and open the mind to create space for fresh ways to live life. Engage in forms of meditation that create erect posture allowing easy access to our minds eye. Wander through a park or trek along a beautiful beach to access the mind's eye. Switch the radio off in the car and leave the TV off at night. Rid our surroundings of all distractions and tune in to the limitless possibilities we possess within. Let our creative mind understand, deeply and intuitively.

PERCEPTIVE SENSE

Who we become and what we see is determined by our perception. Our experience of life reflects our perceptual viewpoint, which stems from our level of awareness. In essence, *our interpretation* of things *creates our experience.* Life's events are the outcome of our own choices, beliefs, and goals. In reality, truth is subjective, what we believe we see, we think to be true. The key is to dethrone our mind from its tyranny as being the sole arbiter of reality through creative leaps of awareness. This way we evolve our sense of perception to take in a wider perspective of life.

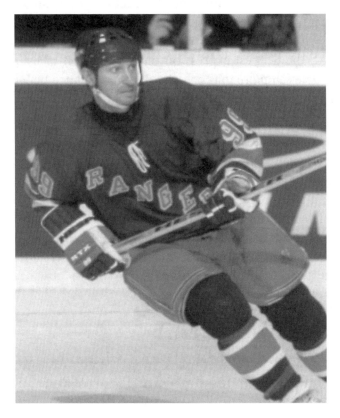

Wayne Gretzky cultivated the power to harness the inner reality to perceive the flow of things, without thought.

Our mind experiences our experience. The mind however in the process, by its very nature try's to convince us that our unique point of view is the genuine reality. The first step to expanding our level of awareness is to surrender the notion that "I know". When we *free our mind* from accepting that our learned behavior is the only way to view things, and acknowledge that not everything needs to be intellectualized, we open the gateway to sense life beyond logic. Our perceptive sense is what keeps us *in the flow of life* as it occurs around us. The initial step is to *harness our inner reality first*, only then can we begin to sense in a more perceptive manner, from moment to moment the reality of what is really happening?

The *power of perception* enables us to manifest in life what others call genius. Take the example of ice hockey great, Wayne Gretzgy, "most people chase the puck, I go where the puck is going to be." He'd mastered the art of moving effortlessly into an empty space, as if he knew instinctively where to be at precisely the right instant to receive the puck and score. Martial artists train for years to master the same technique, to *be at one with the environment*, to move in-synch with the flow of their opponent, aware of their intentions. They see life in fluid-motion-time, as opposed to static-motion-time, and this gives them the edge in combat and sport. The power to *perceive the flow of things* is to see or know it as we do it, without thought. Power and perception go hand in hand

Bodies talk to bodies. We not only communicate through spoken language, we also communicate through body language. When we learn to *trust what we sense and feel*, we open up to a whole new world of tactile communication and information. The *wisdom of our body* orchestrates our natural thinking and behavioral flow in life. Relying on thinking alone traps us into our learned behavior, where we see, think and respond in fixed ways.

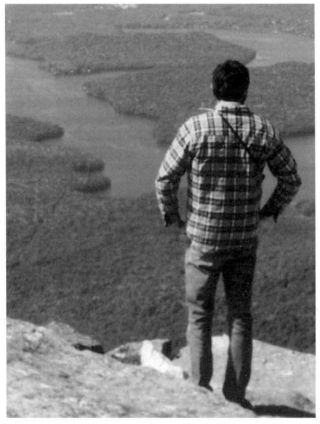

Conceptualize through the power of vision,
and feel the essence of what we want
as an impulse in our heart.

Often our perception is just a piece of reality's pie, not the whole thing. We're not robots, we possess a body of knowledge with the power of perception to sense beyond the realms of logic. To intuitively be in touch with the flow of things, we need to listen to our body and sense what to do. The logic of life then becomes apparent.

For any real personal transformation to manifest, our idea of the body and the way we relate to the world has to shift. Focusing our *minds awareness* into our belly merges thinking with feeling creating a more holistic approach. Life feels and looks different when we unite senses with reason. We can't always trust what we think we see. Assumption is the mother of illusion. Best to sharpen our sense of perception.

PERSONAL VISION

We are more than we have become. Our ability to envisage an epic journey that a thousand words could not begin to describe, is our access to life's infinite field of potentiality. Our pathway to realize our true potential emerges from our capacity to *see what our heart feels*. The lifetime opportunity to align and express our unique creative self.

Each of us possesses a *god given talent*, a blueprint to a potentially successful life. We first gain insight to our talents as a young kid. If we were lucky enough to be guided by our parents, teachers or relatives whom recognized our natural born talents, we developed them. If we were in tune with them our self, and followed our inner voice, chances are we're on our true path, living our dream. If we didn't chances are life has become somewhat of an act, living out someone else's dream, an unsatisfactory existence. The good news is that a journey can change direction at any

FEARLESS SPIRIT, JOYOUS HEART

time, the one we want be on is the one that's aligned to us. The future we see defines the person we become.

To access our personal vision, we need to *tune in* and listen to what our deeper parts are calling us to be. The things in life that stretch who we are and draw out our creative self, whilst bringing us fulfillment, and the feeling of having a natural flair. Our unique talents are our gifts to society, and they are our responsibility to unleash. There are many vocations in life, not all of them at first appear logical or practical in terms of generating happiness or money. People will advise us to get a real job, one that offers security and a future; some may even choose a career path for us. The real question is *what is our passion*. What lights our fire and urges us to pour our soul into life. If our work brings us joy, then we're on the path to unleashing creative talents. Each of us can have a rich life, doing what we love with passion, when we believe in what our heart sees.

The true person blocking our vision is inevitably our self. Nobody makes us choose our path in life. Others may influence us, but we alone must harness the spirit to stand our ground with the hearts courage to pursue our dreams. Our vision is the magnet pulling us towards what we can become. My mother used to say to me; "*if you don't wake up with a smile on your face you must be doing something wrong*"? Nothing in our life is more important than following our hearts path with all our spirit, to *live our dream.*

We each have something to *contribute* during our lifetime. When we embrace our true talents, we see how our actions can benefit all people. Without fulfillment, we lose our heart and spirit. Life becomes empty and meaningless. Following our dream will test us, we'll need to stay fearless in our quest and maintain the ability to laugh at our mistakes or misfortunes along the way. Never let anyone tell us it can't be done. Always *think big.*

Nothing in life just happens, our success is dependent upon our efforts. Everything rides on the tip of our motivation, which ultimately comes from our *courage to live our truths with passion.* Life presents opportunities and doors will open, but there are no guarantees, only chances. We alone get to choose if we'll keep our minds eye focused on what we want at all times, and our perception keen. A moment's deviation can mean the difference between dreaming, and awakening to live the dream.

SURFING THE EDGE

Life is a journey, a series of events that create our future. We move towards more powerful realms by entertaining more creative performance levels. By concentrating our thoughts beyond our current ability. By visualizing the person we wish to be and the things we aim to do. Through cultivating a *free flowing* meditative *mind-set* for life, each moment is like surfing the edge of what can be. In life, free the mind to see what's possible and *go to the limits* of our choice.

In all biological systems growth comes from the periphery. At *the edge* of our current ability lurks the opportunity for immense growth. Life's luck is found at the perimeter of our present potential, which means we need to constantly *challenge our self.* We must extend our self and be prepared to live a little outside our comfort zone. Quitting too soon, when the going gets tough means we become despondent and abandon our efforts. In times of difficulty we need to persevere. Once we commit to a cause, the universe will test us. If our heart is true and our spirit strong, we will begin to see our efforts being rewarded through creative insights that become *opportunities for growth.* Each time we bring our heart and soul to what we do, we cultivate the energy to see things in new ways.

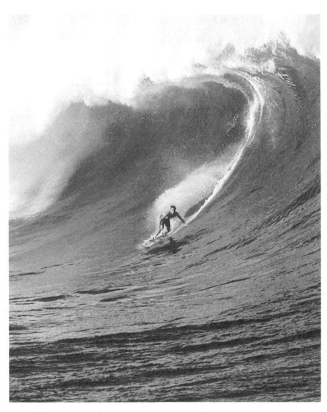

Like surfing, life challenges us to journey beyond the edge of our comfort zones. To free the mind, see what's possible and go for it.

Innovation is creative *visionary thinking*. It is our impetus for growth, originating from our imagination. Our ability to see and think outside the square is an invisible power able to generate limitless possibilities. The majority of successful people in the world started with an idea, a vision. The computer, music, video and sporting worlds are testimony to this where 15 years ago making serious money and living happy in these fields were just a dream. To access the minds power of imagination is to *free the mind* from its learned behavior and habitual responses. In this way we learn to expand our energy and develop our conscious way of thinking to allow new ways of responding to circumstances to enter into our life. Retain a *beginner's mind*, free from limitations and boundaries. Open up to receiving and perceiving a constant flow of possibilities in life.

Thoughts run through our whole body or as the eastern sages remind us; *thought is concentrated body energy*. When we allow our awareness to sink into the gravitational center of our body, 1-2 inches below our navel, we create an inner calmness that opens our mind and allows our senses to flow. This inner power is what martial artists call *the body's eye*, the home of our *intuitive power*. It's from here the surfer instinctively rides with the flow of the wave. With a sense of what's ahead we can create a strategy, with a feeling of flow to live in a more creative way.

Being centered enables us to view life from a *point of observation*. Our whole being becomes aware of thinking, feeling and sensing in new ways. It develops *big picture thinking*, the capacity to look beyond a problem to possible solutions. This necessitates a mind-set of detachment from the problem to make way for a solution. Rather than thinking about our problems, be free to concentrate on what our solutions are. The power to focus beyond obstacles is what brings creativity to our life. From this experience the fluidity and sense of direction is thorough and inventive.

SOUL KEYS

*We choose what we create - Tune to the positive
and take ownership of this life*

*Our creative mind is our magic wand -
Whatever we visualize or imagine we invite into
our life - The key question is what do we want?*

*Who we become and what we see is
determined by our perception - Through creative
leaps of awareness we evolve our sense of
perception to take in a wider view of life*

*What lights our fire and urges us to
pour our soul   into life? -
Have the courage to live our truths
with passion - be our dream*

*Free the mind to see what's possible
and go to the limits of our choice*

CHAPTER 3

THE WILL TO ACT

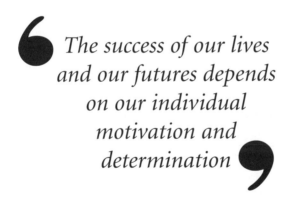

The success of our lives and our futures depends on our individual motivation and determination

THE DALAI LAMA

WILLPOWER

When mountaineers attempt a peak, the more hardship they endure along the way, the greater the joy they feel on reaching the summit. The challenge itself continuously pushes them beyond their comfort zone as the question is asked of them; How determined are they to move forward and reach their goal? To succeed they must draw on every ounce of their *inner resolve*. The risk of temporarily losing a foothold is far outweighed by the risk of losing the opportunity of a lifetime. The *self-initiated effort* we make to stay on course is what *propels our journey* towards our intended destination.

Willpower requires *concentration* on the task at hand. It is the ability to focus our mind, and deliver on our intention. We are often limited by our mind's reluctance to focus beyond its current power. The *will to persevere* comes when we can identify our resistance to something or acknowledge our self-defeating patterns of thoughts and behaviors. Life without the will to take action is time lost forever. Our willpower is the tool of our mind to win this eternal battle. It is the difference between talking the talk and walking the walk. The will to act lays the foundation for everything we do in life.

The mind's inclination is *towards pleasure* and *away from pain*. This focus distracts us from the present moment and diminishes our power to concentrate our will. Either way we lose *the power of the moment*. The potency of our willpower is determined by our ability to stay focused on the process, to identify what needs to be done, and do it. The key is to bring our choices to the level of conscious awareness, so that our actions align to our goals. Anything less is too weak to make us strong. Through strength of mind our body comes to know what has to be done. The will to do more, steady as we go, with patience, one step at a time towards

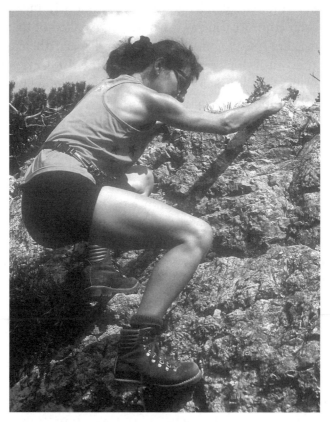

*The self-initiated effort we make to stay on course
is what propels our journey towards our intended
destination.*

our goal. The power to stay focused in the moment with the end goal in mind, breathe and give it our all.

We must *will our self*. When the going gets tough, the brave look to the strength of their heart and spirit. Taking action in the face of fear and at the expense of our ego, makes the difficult seem easy and the impossible attainable. Our *sense of fearlessness* juxtaposed with our *hearts courage* empowers our mind and body. Fearless Spirit, Joyous Heart contains the essence of willpower. The attitude of absorbing our self *whole-heartedly* into what we do with spirited determination and immense passion.

Iron willpower comes through bodily experience. Engaging in a *physical practice* like running, yoga or martial arts is what integrates and reinforces *new patterns* of thought and behavior necessary for lasting change. Physical participation reveals our inner brokenness, our limitations and weaknesses of character from which we can't escape. Physical practice builds an inner confidence that strengthens our state of mind and body. This strengthens our *will to act*. To follow through and experience small victories, which give us the fortitude to endure and press on.

The choices we make require *sacrifices*; that is the test. To deliver on our intentions is to visualize our objective, focus our mind and willfully make our thoughts reality. Without *focused feeling* and *dedication* our desires remain wishful thinking

SETTING THE MIND

Martial arts speak of *setting the mind*. Hours are spent training to detach and stay calm amidst the chaos of battle or life. The psychological war regardless of situation starts within. This occurs by accessing a *centered state* that allows our intuitive wisdom and precise timing to lead the way. When a warrior loses *internal balance* their opponent can then dictate their actions.

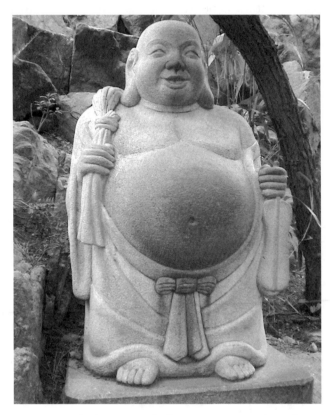

*By quieting our mind, we create a point of
attention, a still point, with the enhanced
clarity to perceive past the inflexible
nature of habit and thought*

Warriors understand that victory demands composure, patience and the will to attain the correct mind-set to direct their power. With the right action, comes victory.

The mind is circular and affirming. What we anticipate our mind searches for, it follows our expectations and searches out those things, which confirm and conform to our beliefs. In essence, life becomes a self-fulfilling experience, as we make our mind believe that there is little possibility for anything else. The *beginners mind*, keeping a *freshness of inquiry*, is what enhances our ability to make the right choices in life. By quieting our mind, we create a point of attention, a "still point", with the enhanced clarity to perceive past the inflexible nature of habit and thought. This way our mind remains clear, able to link the center of our experience with the core of our body, to instinctively respond to the world around us. We transcend beyond the boundary of mind set through our habits established in past experience, and through our expectations. *Life is a field of potentiality*. From stillness, we open our mind to possibilities, and allow our *intuitive self* to be the creative choice maker.

Deep within is an *inner voice*, our internal guide to what is right for us. What we know as going with our gut instinct, or seizing an opportunity placed before us. It *just feels right*. To obtain this mind-set, try detaching from anticipating the outcome, and simply respond, just act. This requires the willpower to listen and flow with the wisdom of our body, and instinctively approach any human endeavor for what it is. Rather than manufacture life, *simply let it unfold.* Our *intuitive mind* guides us when we are stuck. We have the choice to follow its lead. Trust what we sense and feel as our response. The deepest part of us yearns to live true to our self.

To set our mind, imagine sitting in *the eye of a hurricane* with an empty mind and alert body. Now focus on the breath, this is the key to synchronizing body and mind to broaden our point of observation. When we stop to question and judge our circumstances, our mind starts to think, and in that moment we detach from what we were actually experiencing. When our mind is correctly calibrated we instinctively sense an outward flow from deep in our core as to what to do in that moment. Our ability to access knowledge from a place of *inner calm* and *clarity* enables us to handle what life throws at us with "effortless effort". A developed will, which lives beyond ego and simply flows.

The key is to keep our mind as still as a mountain at all times. To meditate our awareness upon where we are now, whilst being conscious of our thoughts and feelings, which determine our actions. To achieve the mental clarity and emotional stability to act in the present moment, firstly focus our breath in our *lower abdomen.* This is our body's gravitational center where we anchor our actions. Secondly concentrate our mind *between our eyebrows,* the physical seat of our will. The more we focus, that is, enliven what the mystics call our *luminous essence,* the more powerful our *intuitive will* becomes. The more we resonate to be at one with life.

SELF-AWARENESS

We are what we think we are, what others think we are and what we really are. In life, there is often a disparity between the way things appear to us and the way they actually are. Awareness expands our *conscious presence.* We become more mindful of every action with the assurance of the truth of each experience. Self-awareness allows us to interact with the world in a more authentic manner.

Each day we awaken to our most dominant beliefs. We are

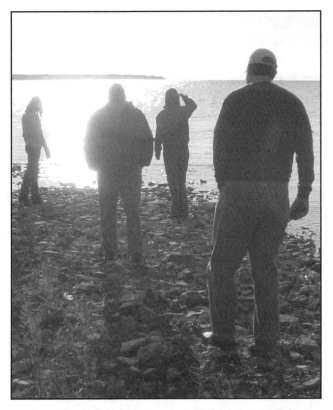

*We are what we think we are, what others think we
are and what we really are.*

creatures of habit, and our thoughts will us into action. Often what we think we're doing in life and what we're actually doing are two different things. The first and most important step to becoming who we want to be in life is the awareness of who we are now. We must *live fully* in the moment, know our thoughts, choose our words and align our actions with our goals.

The first step to awareness is to *notice the truth about where we sit* in the scheme of things. We are a manifestation of our most dominant habits. The fundamental question is whether our current behavior is moving us towards our dreams. To identify the power of our habitual actions, stop and acknowledge current patterns of behavior. The least productive is *unconscious awareness*, where we're controlled by our compulsions, obsessions, habits, addictions and attachments. Next is *conscious awareness*, where we're aware of our inappropriate behaviors but not yet ready to take responsibility. Then there's *conscious awareness* and *action*, where we begin to operate from self-responsibility with the acceptance that our actions create our life. Ultimately we're aiming for *total awareness*, the state whereby we're mindfully aware of the intuitive wisdom that calls us to act, whilst having awareness of all our actions with integrity and responsibility. As the saying goes, "beyond illusion is insight". The key in this process to self-mastery is to *pause* and *reflect* with self-awareness, possess the willpower to change, align our goals with reality and have the discipline to direct our actions towards our goals.

Self-awareness allows us to *examine the nature of our beliefs*. Beliefs form our thought structure, which influence the choices we make and the life we experience. Any idea we accept as truth becomes a belief that forms a part of our reality. Our progress begins when we realize the only time we can make a difference and actually live reality is *right here and right now*. Awareness means being objective about whether our current beliefs contribute towards the growth of our character. It is necessary to possess the will to replace redundant beliefs by *shifting our thinking* to create and live our ideal reality. The only beliefs we want are those that move us towards becoming a better person in all walks of life. Self-awareness is akin to moving like the fox that observes every little distraction of thought and adjusts its plan of action accordingly.

The practice of *self-awareness* is the *vehicle for change*. When our behavior aligns with our goals, we are ensured success where willpower alone has failed. Take the example of exercising to change our body shape. We can train like a beast possessed, but unless our training regime is structured correctly, our eating plan is healthy enough to build a resilient body and we facilitate adequate recovery, we will fail to make the progress we deserve, despite our headstrong will to succeed. The key is to focus on what brings success.

INDOMITABLE SPIRIT

To succeed in life is to learn to engage. To be prepared to give our all. Key is having the invincible power to use the *mind as a generator*, not as a reactor. To harness the *indomitable spirit* means energizing our self with the will to *create positive effects*.

Life is full of challenging situations that require willpower to overcome. Learning not to overreact emotionally affords us the clarity to generate favorable solutions. When we bring our intent into the present moment, we maintain conscious awareness of our thoughts and words. In doing so we avoid being hooked into agendas and the fears of others. We remain free to align our mind to our inner and outer worlds. Though our intent may be noble, our flesh at times weakens. Life demands spirit, there is no hope for a coward. Cultivate a *brave heart* and *strong mind* to successfully move forward in life.

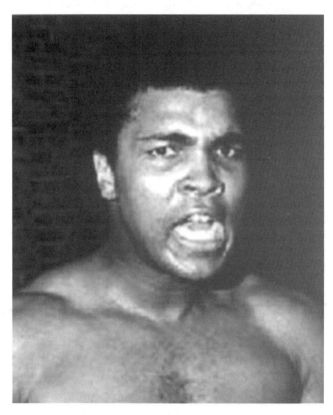

Muhammad Ali had the courage to say, "I don't have to be who you want me to be"; "I'm fighting for my freedom". We each have the free will to become the embodiment of what we want to be in the world.

Our mind is home to creative *thoughts*. Our *emotions* are the bridge between mind and body. Together they are the *causes* and *effects* of our life. They determine the intent of our actions or the way we respond to events. Everything we do starts with a single thought that determines the direction of our attention. This is followed by an emotion that determines the charge our actions carry. Emotionally charged thoughts become magnetic and attract similar thoughts, that then manifest exponentially. Repetitive negative thoughts become destructive whereas repetitive positive thoughts become constructive. We are the only person who can think in our mind. To live life fully, *master our mind* to engage with an *indomitable spirit*, show up and *give our best*.

Life is a reflection of our inner world. How *balanced* and *resilient* we've become on the inside to manage the external forces of life we encounter. Each day is full of circumstances that test our mettle. We see if we have the *heart to fight* for what we believe in, the *will to succeed* in the face of opposition, the capacity to relentlessly pursue our goals regardless of what happens. We must strive to keep our internal focus and *never surrender* our mind to others, instead continuing to do what needs to be done. When our competitive spirit becomes a conscious part of our thinking and speaking, our thoughts and words stay positive and uplifting even in situations of discord. Our actions are constructive and appropriate. Right action follows right thinking.

Engaging with awareness makes the difference. Our capacity to *put our heart into action*, with constant attention to our thinking, the words we use, and the feelings we entertain. Fundamentally our thought process determines our actions. Our ability to *pause and consider* the effect of our actions on our self and others, determines whether we align our inner and outer worlds. Remember, reputation precedes action. The need to be true to our self and work our butts off is a reality. Life demands that we pay our dues.

Understanding theory alone is useless. Everything must be *continuously practiced* so that it becomes an unconscious part of our thought process. Our intent and will synthesize our inner and outer worlds. With clear intention our actions are already half completed. All we have to do is commit, follow through and give it form and polish.

FREE WILL

We are born with an innately *curious nature* - to explore the adventures that lay before us, the unknown. The very essence of our being desires the *freedom to experience* as much of life as possible. The limits we place upon ourselves inhibit our will to participate fully in life with an *adventurous spirit*. Our mind directs our willpower and must be free to flow with the nature of things, like an inquisitive bird that flies to its heart's content.

Where there's free will there's a way. Each of us has the power to make the decisions that *shape our future*. The only person who can motivate us in life is our self. Others may inspire us but the will to succeed comes from our ability to accept that *our own power is our creator*. Life is too short to merely echo other people's expectations and live a life that's not original. When we're not attached to what others think about us, we're more capable of expressing our true self and speaking our mind freely. Those who embrace chances in life, take the attitude that this is my life and I will use my free will to think and feel as I see best. We are all free to *express our will* to live the life we choose. All we have to do is let our inquisitive nature run free.

Our *mind is our power*. It is up to us to use it well. When our mind is scattered, we lack the discipline to see a task through to completion. When our mind is rigid, we lack the awareness to see the opportunities that are before us. As the Tai Chi saying goes, "Too little is the same as too much". Our *mind must be free* to *adapt and change* with the nature of things. An open mind is free to relinquish that which no longer serves our growth, to admit that which will empower us to create a life in alignment with our heart.

Someone once said that the world belongs to the brave. Those who are prepared to *name and claim* what it is they want in life. Possessing free will means having the *freedom to choose* what's acceptable and what's not acceptable in our life. It's the power to set the boundaries as to what we will let in and what we will keep out. Grab a pen and draw a circle on a piece of paper. On the inside write all the things you will accept in your life and around the outside write all the things you wish to omit. Use this as your *power statement* to the world conveying who you are and what your will is to others at a subconscious level. Don't compromise your life. Claiming back our *sense of self* empowers us to live free.

We have *the choice to step up* and claim our life or to sit back and watch time tick away. The ability to work hard is the foundation to support our talents. We can't rest on our laurels, we've got to do the hard yards and make things happen. Understand that *our progress in life is based on our own efforts*. To rely on someone else for success, only weakens our ability to create our own life. The victory for willpower tests our *strength of spirit* and *hearts resolve* to be decisive and persevere. Remember, being impatient in trivial matters seldom enables us to achieve success in matters of great importance. As Boxing legend Muhammad Ali put it best "float like a butterfly and sting like a bee". Let the mind dance with life, make decisions seamlessly and take action with the utmost sincerity. Live Free, Be Self.

SOUL KEYS

*The self-initiated effort we make
to stay on course is what propels our journey
towards our intended destination*

*The beginners mind, keeping a freshness
of inquiry, is what enhances our ability
to make the right choices in life*

*Self-awareness expands our
conscious presence to notice the truth
about where we sit in the scheme of things*

*Use the mind as a generator
to harness the indomitable spirit
to create positive effects*

*To accept our own power as our creator –
we must be willing to name
and claim what we want*

CHAPTER 4

EXPERIENCE WHOLENESS

The spirit in thee is a river.
Its sacred bathing place is contemplation;
Its waters are truth;
Its banks are holiness;
Its waves are love.
Go to the river for purification:
Thy soul cannot be made pure
by mere water

THE BHAGAVAD GITA

CENTERING

*The aim is a state of stillness and clarity,
a level of consciousness that awakens a
deeper awareness of our true self.*

*Sit either on the floor, a mat or in a chair
with your back erect, body relaxed, eyes
and mouth closed. Now, bring your attention
to your breath and enter silence.*

*As you inhale, gently allow your belly to rise,
then your chest to expand*

*As you exhale, naturally allow your
chest to relax, then your belly to contract.*

*Be conscious only of your breath, fully aware
of the space between the inhalation and
exhalation. Let the experience unfold
spontaneously like the flow of water in a river.*

*The key is diligent practice; start with 5 minutes
daily. As the mind becomes calmer, prolong to 30
minutes. When we center our energy, our intellect
sharpens, our mental strength toughens and our
power of compassion heightens. Only then can we
begin to master our world.*

Ancient cultures honored the body as an alchemical entity. They believed when energy flowed correctly within the body it created an *alchemical transformation* manifesting wholeness. The laws dictated that the energy of life moved in a circle, in a perfect flow of balance. It was believed that until one discovered their center, their circle would never be complete, and that they would never know wholeness. Our center is our *vortex of energy*. The place from where our true nature radiates into the various aspects of life. From here we *experience embodiment* and dance to the beat of our own drum.

Our body is the house we inhabit. To make authentic changes in our life we have to *center our energy flow*. We have to journey beneath layers of awareness and descend into our core. To the home of our real essence, *the soul of our being*. It is here we find our true self, inscribed with inherent gifts and talents that interconnect us with the web of life. By concentrating our awareness about our navel we center our energy. This fosters the spontaneous flow of our true nature from our core, out through our body and into the world. This *process of expansion* expresses all that we are whilst maintaining contact with our true integrity. The quest for our center is *the journey of awareness*, the path towards unfolding the true destiny within us. Living from the soul.

Obtaining wholeness is like undertaking the journey of putting *humpty dumpty back together* again. It is something we must experience first hand and arrive at our self. The more we connect with our center, the clearer we begin to see life from the inside looking out. Our body is the *seat of our liberation*, the primary *anchor of our awareness* that shatters the shell of our conditioning to sense our true journey within us that longs to experience completeness. We unify the totality of our being. Like a spider spinning a web from its center, we too can venture out to experience everything with true wholeness.

About the navel is our center. Like the hub of a wheel or the axle of a propeller, energy in motion becomes fluid from its point of balance. Our center is the *communication hub* of our body. Here we merge reason and instinct to know that our actions are aligned with our highest aspirations. To locate our *center of power* position both hands *1-2 inches below the navel,* take a deep breath in and exhale fully, then laugh like the Buddha with his big smiling belly. The contracting muscles felt beneath the hands is the place of power where consolidation of wholeness naturally occurs. Activities such as martial arts, sport,yoga, pilates, meditation, painting, sculpting, singing and dancing awaken our center.

Centering anchors our experience. It enhances our energy-flow, mimicking the ripple effect of a pebble thrown into a pond. We create the still-point from which soul and self are encircled, and accentuate our power to move closer to a soulful life. To *live centered,* connect mind to breath and breath to center. Breath is the core of life, the thread weaving us together to experience our self as *one power* from a place of inner stillness. Here consciousness, awareness and manifestation merge. In reality, life is intricately mysterious and ultimately incomprehensible to rational ways of thinking. Centered, we integrate mind, body and spirit to live a deeply rich, and satisfying life.

LIVE HERE AND NOW

What happens here and now, determines the future. Being centered enhances our conscious presence to live the truth of now, towards our future. Self-awareness is the initial link, in our quest to live *fully present,* in the eternal moment of *here and now.*

Life is happening now. Each event comprises of the *inner realm* of our thoughts, and the *outer realm* of our environment. To

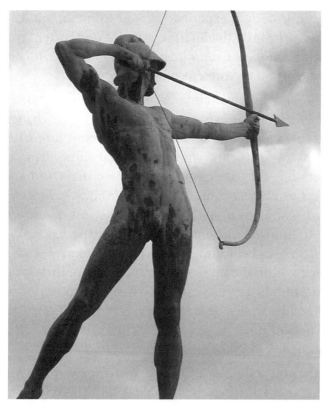

*Employing the essence of all we are into what we do
impels our soul into life.*

become *one* with the flow of life and align our behavior with the present, there can be no body-mind split. We must experience life as a whole being using all our senses, and focus now. When we see past the illusion of what our mind conceives, we *experience reality*. We become fully mindful of our *doing* and *being*. By tuning into what our body is experiencing, our thinking mind and feeling body synchronize the interpretation of our current reality. We manifest the *stillness within activity* that enables us to instantly intuit the truth of the present moment.

Life is not an outer circumstance but an inner experience. It is a *way of being* that exists independently of our changing fortunes. At the center of our being we gather information on a non-intellectual level. Like the smile of joy that shines from our eyes demonstrating the contentment our *belly feels* and our *heart knows*. Self-awareness comes through our body. It flows from our belly's gut awareness up into our heart, the seat of our emotions, onward to inform our intellect of our experience. When we breathe from our belly and keep our mind on our breath we center our self within the present moment. Our bodily response now leads our minds representation. When we come to *trust our instincts* and let things be, less becomes more. All our senses step into the flow of now.

Our belly is home to our *inner awareness*. Being centered we possess the power to *relax* and *merge* with everyday life. The yielding principle is nature's way of dealing with the unyielding. This interplay of forces requires us to *stay centered* as we adapt and change with life's events and still hold it all together. To be in it: but not of it. To be fully present in the here and now and spontaneously interact with the circumstance as befits the situation. Everybody reacts to life differently. It is our response that counts, not the event itself. We master our actions by using our center as the point of reference to view life from a place of *inner calmness*

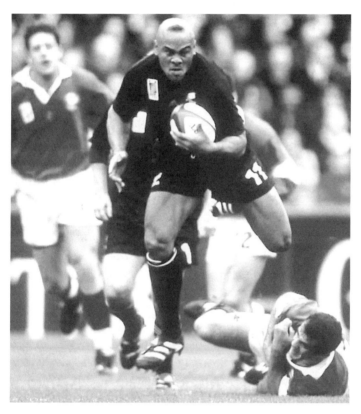

The time to start living life is now.
This moment is our life.

with an *alert awareness* of the present moment. Living our experiences in our body, embraces the motto, live for tomorrow, mindfully today.

Centering saves us from becoming disembodied. When we seek refuge from reality, with a life that remains a fantasy of thoughts inside our mind of a future that never actually happens, we live imprisoned in an illusion. We separate our self from our body. Our body is our vehicle for self-awakening. By centering our energy, our whole being starts to think, feel and be, all at the same time. We *embody the full awareness of our actual experience.* This awakens us from the illusion to enlighten our mind, that in reality, we are our experiences.We exist as a matrix of energy and information, with our body the storehouse of knowledge, our life history, and our head the viewing screen. Engaging our body in life is the key. Every experience is a *lesson in wisdom,* each one becomes a part of us at our soul level. The *act of doing* breaks through our fears to live in the here and now, *the real thing,* to fulfill our potential. We experience life *firsthand.* Learn to trust our instincts, because they link our now to embody our future.

LET LIFE FLOW

The metaphor of flowing water is often paralleled to the image of life. Water is in a constant state of flux. Waters diverse ability to be both assertive and yielding is what gives it the possibility to *flow with the nature of things* and utilize its power. Our lives are a flow of constantly changing experiences that require a sense of life's shifting times. The inherent rhythms to dance with what comes, and fearlessly *let go* to experience the truth of who we are.

Life's events have an *energy flow.* To position our self with

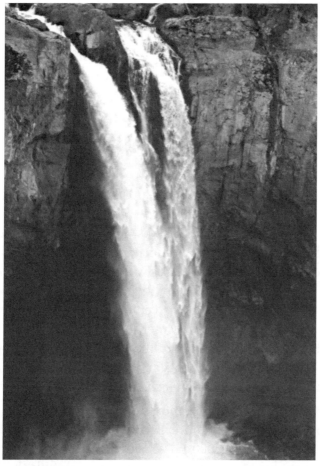

Water has the power to flow with the nature of things. Our true self is always in motion like the river of life, constantly changing.

the flow of things in life we need to create our own *center of flow*. The intuitive place we gather our *sense of awareness* to harness the *stream of consciousness* to instinctively respond amidst any situation. By centering our attention we encompass our thinking and feeling states to coordinate the appropriate response. This affords us internal focus, while simultaneously absorbing with sensitivity the flow of life around us. We're able to let slide thoughts and emotions that could throw us off-center and scatter our energy. Establishing our *sense of center* as we interact in the world, directs our energy flow in a more *creative direction*. We harness the state of mind that observes the moment, unfolds from within and flows.

Life flow revels in *fluidity* and *flexibility*. When we remain rigid in our beliefs and actions we limit our options in life. The most harmonious human actions echo the patterns found in nature. Depending on our circumstances we should be able to be as hard as a diamond, flexible as a willow, smooth as flowing water or as empty as space. The ability to *relax and merge* with the essence of things whilst staying centered within the vortex of our power. When we lose our center, our sense of timing to flow melodically with the nature of things diminishes. With our mind set in our center, our thoughts and actions unite and our stream of consciousness comes *on line* instinctively.

Our energy flows harmoniously when we gather information on a *sensory level* and experience life from *home base,* our center. The seat of structural sensitivity, from where our kinesthetic sense for life accumulates and every cell feels the integrity of our actions. Centered, we gain a clearer perspective of our self and a wider perspective of life. We literally "pull our self together" to generate gut instinct in any given moment. Our instincts represent our *spontaneous power* to *unleash our creative juices* and flow with what we experience. In this state of being, our body does the thinking, and our mind dances with life. Our center is our *instinctive compass* and from here we navigate life.

Life is a continuum with our *body and mind intricately wired* to change. Our mind entertains a field of ideas that it thinks about subjectively. Our body entertains a field of *molecules of emotions* that it experiences objectively. Wherever our thoughts go, molecules go, and our brain is in a perpetual flux, reflecting moment to moment our changing experiences. Our body is the storehouse of our *feelings*. They are the language that links our entire being. Our potential to live life in a fluid-like manner is realized when we embrace our mental, physical and emotional. As the saying goes, "a part is never as strong as the whole, balance is the key". Become mindful of staying centered.

EMPOWER SELF

Our intentions create our experiences. They either tear us apart or make us stronger and more whole as a person. Our biggest challenge to overcome in life is our own barrage of opposing thoughts. One part of us says one thing and another says something else. When we pull our self together, so to speak, we empower our self to *accept responsibility* for our future through *acts of power.*

Empowering our center empowers our life. Coaching externally with high intensity yelling and ego-stroking "rah-rah" like some motivational speakers do to a room full of hysterical people gives a false sense of self. It's only a matter of time before our ego's imaginary wall of invincibility crumbles away, and depression and a sense of loss returns. Our real power is inside us. We must *make the shift within first.* The choice is between our ego and our true self. To exist immersed in ego is to live a restricted, imprisoned life. Our ego is our superficial social mask that thrives on approval

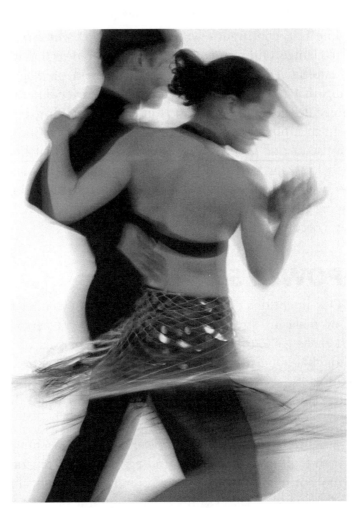

The body speaks the language of the soul.
It is our vehicle for life.

and control. Centering resonates an awareness of our true sense of self. We become more conscious of our intuitive power, urging us to bring more soul, authenticity, to empower our personality. Trust the assurance and serenity that emanates from within, and follow this as our strategy in life.

Self-power comes through the physical act of facing our self. Having the *courage* and *spontaneity* to do what resonates deep inside us. Without soulful action life is just talk, and thoughts. We empower our self through engaging in life. Each success we come to know, builds our self-esteem and confidence towards what we can accomplish in life. Our power to take action comes from the *internal framework* we build around our center where we balance logic and feeling. It does not originate from our ego with its protective shields of armor that hide our true feelings. The power of inner strength makes us less defensive about who we are, much freer to experience and express all that we are.

Being centered *harnesses our power*. Martial artists, dancers and athletes know peak performance relies on supporting their entire being about their center. When our concentration turns inward to gel our mind's intellect with our body's instinct, authentic acts of power become our natural response. They just feel right. This illustrates where the true strength of our character resides and the wholeness of our being gathers. Through wholeness, every cell in our body has the power to overcome the perceived self-made fears that stand in our way. We empower our self with the *backbone to commit* to our endeavors. We never then have to entertain the thoughts – "If only I had" or "What if!"

Many people are jolted toward their true journey in the face of tragedy or when illness strikes. When we realize every event is a catalyst to bringing a deeper awareness of our state of affairs we can use this to realign to our purpose. We can use our intelligence and choose to *act positively*. Do not hold back, life is far too short, *welcome every moment* as an opportunity of self-dis-covery to the exploration of wholeness. We are our own *pattern of energy flow*, the habitual way we view and grasp the world. As a famous Chinese Philosopher once said, "grasshopper, we express power by choice, focus and direct with responsibility". We realize we can succeed when we acknowledge that time is the essence of life, and that *time is our doing*. Remember we don't have to be per-fect; life is a process.

BE AUTHENTIC

There is an old Indian saying that explains the interrela-tionship of mass, energy and experiences; "To know a persons experiences from the past examine their body now. To know a persons body in the future, examine their experiences now". We are shaped by our actions. In reality, we've got to *become the change* we want to see in the world.

Success in life and as a person is *something we become*. It is not something we achieve. Our perceptions create our reality and our beliefs create our biology. The *true index* to how our journey is progressing in life is our body. The mind knows how to lie, as it creates illusions to protect the ego. The body resonates to us what it knows is best. It is our reality check. The body speaks *the lan-guage of our soul* and is the vehicle for the inner transformation that's not possible solely through an intellectual process. To become the embodiment of our goals, we must begin with the end in mind. Then *work on the process* of becoming all the things we need to be. The key is to *focus on the impulses* that fuelled the ini-tial passion we had for our dreams. Keep asking, what resonates?

Being authentic requires us to *know our self*. Not just our strengths, but to coax, or even dare the parts of us that aren't our strengths into action. The simple act of walking through our fears is what liberates us from self-bondage to self-power. Our state of being whereby we *remain centered*, and grounded to reality, with the good sense to accept life's challenges. Being authentic is not to dance to someone else's beat. It is to live in harmony with the rhythm of our own soul's resonating song. What we know in our heart and guts to be us. When we drop the limitations of our ego and embrace the unlimited consciousness that resides within us, our thinking evolves to a more creative way of *being* and our behavior to a more authentic way of *doing*. Our physical experience of life is then attuned to harnessing all our energy to *create* a *soulful life.*

Life presents us with opportunities to realize our full potential. Our ability to *claim our power* and not let others take away our sense of self is crucial. Life becomes laced with tragedy when we allow others to manipulate our thoughts and actions. We literally give them permission to control the outcomes in our life. The only way we move towards fulfilling our dreams is to *stay true* to our self. Centering our energy we learn to *trust our feelings*, honor what makes our *heart pound*, and take authentic action. Life is about being who we are. There is honor in this way. Belief in our self is imperative to staying on track to the creative experience of living all that we are.

Being authentic is living true to our heart, and performing up to our capabilities. Our *choices* make us who we are today. They are our future. Every choice has its consequences. We become enslaved or empowered, feel empty or consolidated. We learn to *live our truth by trusting our heart* in the brief moment it speaks to us. Before our mind has time to reason an alternative. Our actions, when aligned towards our highest growth become building blocks. They assemble our sense of wholeness to speak and take action from our instinctive core. It is the person we are inside that really matters. At the end of the day we must live with our self.

SOUL KEYS

Our navel is our vortex of energy
from where we center our self with
the awareness of the soul of our being

Centered we become fully mindful of our
state of doing and being to live fully present,
in the eternal moment of here and now

Our center of flow is the intuitive place we
gather our sense of awareness to harness the
stream of consciousness to instinctively respond
amidst any situation - let life flow

Take responsibility - make the shift to
harness our soul's inner essence - it provides
the backbone to commit to our endeavors

Our body speaks the language of our soul -
live our truth by trusting our heart and
become the change we want to see in the world

CHAPTER 5

THE POSSIBILITIES ARE INFINITE

> *Evolution is a circular process, where we begin with the potential, we fulfil and we go through the process of growth and realize our own true potential*

YOGA SANSKRIT

THE POWER OF LIMITS

There are *no pre-set limits* to what we can experience. Evolution proves there is always more to come. Beyond our current limitations are the doors to an infinite future. The power of limits acts as a force urging us to open these doors in life.

There is a saying, "If you want a new thought, put your body into a new posture". By centering our energy, we shift our way of thinking to a more expanded way of viewing the world. It alters the way we perceive everything. This cultivates the desired state of consciousness that ensures our limitations feed our *creative energy*. Once channeled, we're able *open the inlet* to infinite realms of awareness.

The generative power for *change comes from within.* This is nature's law. From our center of flow, our creative instincts harness our minds eye to delve further into realms of possibility. From our core we begin to question whether or not there is more to life than meets the eye. Our willingness to open our self up to life is key to unlocking doors to new inlets of experience. Authentic *growth unfolds from our core.* Through our capacity to change the way we think and feel, we gain access to more creative realms. This way we continuously evolve through our body and mind, towards living with more conscious awareness. To transcend our limitations, much like the *metamorphosis* of the butterfly, we too can fly freely to our next abode in exploration of life's undiscovered mysteries.

The possibilities are infinite. By centering our energy, our true nature naturally resonates through our solar plexus and heart region. For want of a better term, *the soul of our body*. This expansion is our true self, making its full presence felt, indicating that our state of consciousness has broadened to encompass new levels of awareness. Our quest for infinity begins when we realize; *we are our own limits.*

We have to *go towards limits* to evolve. Our journey is one of courage, where the life we experience is proportionate to the commitment and responsibility we put into our self. We must approach life empty handed and ask questions of everything. The deeper we enquire, the more we realize that a *supreme consciousness* resides within. Our wise, true self, charts our course through life towards a definite goal or purpose. When we center our energy, we navigate our true course by expanding our awareness to new levels of understanding. To evolve, remain *open to the experience* of life. Go to the extremes, and push the boundaries of creation and change.

We are all students of the human race here learning from the school of life. There are two types of students, outer and inner. The outer student learns the various forms, applications and principles of what they do. The inner student studies the craft, the essence of what they do. Seeking guidance from someone with more life experience than we possess, deepens our journey and awakens our creativity. Asking for help is our strength, not our weakness. Find someone who teaches at the heart of life's essence, who sees every lesson as the first lesson. Approach life with *enthusiasm*, this is our source of unlimited energy to transcend our fears and limitations to change our experience of life.

THE WHOLENESS OF BEING

Poetry is the artistic language of the *heart and mind*, symbolic of our capacity to live life as art. To fully engage as it's revealed to us through experience, and still marvel at its mysteries as our understanding deepens. The power to know everything that we are is as every artist's knows, in our soul. Living *openly*

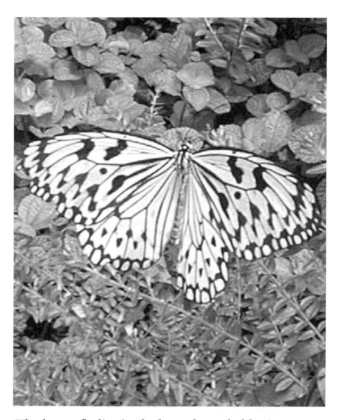

The butterfly lies in darkness bounded by its cocoon and chrysalis, unaware of the light and beauty that waits outside. Once it's completed its metamorphosis, it awakens and breaks free of all limitations to fly free into the realms of the unimaginable.

with courage we complete our wholeness and can live our life as a masterful creation.

Being centered expands our conscious awareness. This concept follows Isaac Newton's *action-reaction* theory, whereby the deeper we resonate from within, the brighter our true nature illuminates forth. This is also supported by the art of meditation, where the action of inner focus prompts the reaction to perceive more expanded realms of awareness. Our center is the *intersection*, where we think our world ends and the rest of the world begins. The origin from where we *align our heart and mind* with our journey. Centering creates the *point of focus* that peels away the layers of illusion and any limiting conceptual thoughts engineered by our mind. Our *body is the storehouse* of our perceptual patterns of energy flow. Changing the way energy flows in our body changes our perception, which is key to changing our life. Opening up enables us to complete our wholeness, and continue to explore the mystery of who we are and our connection to life.

Our spirit inhabits our body. From our center we gain a direct line of communication with what's best for us at any given moment in time. In life, *our body is our teacher*. Listening to our body as it resonates our truth in choosing a certain option or taking a particular path, life feels right. Through merging mind and heart, we become more fluid in our thinking and movement to evolve into our wholeness. This requires the courage to detach from learned ways and live openly and boldly. Trusting what we feel as well as think. Life is about change and whether we can *follow the flow of our spirit* and merge with life's infinite realms of creative experiences.

The *power of discipline* is the foundation to fulfill our potential. It is the difference between avoiding and doing the things that enable us to grow towards more wholeness. When our mind is weak or rigid we become lazy and lack the urgency necessary to live a life with meaning and purpose. Our comfort zone sits inside the status quo and the changing world passes us by. When our mind is centered we access the core of our being, where the *determination to change* resides. Transforming our mind to make genuine lasting change involves our body. The ability to explore what feels right through our body, and to challenge our limitations with *an open mind*. To eliminate the negative we must accentuate the positive, and get on with the things that matter. We must harness the power to open up and unfold to the journey within.

Life demands our *complete involvement*. The totalistic perspective to perceive and make choices that leads to self-realization. The obstacles and constraints we face are in our mind and heart. With the right intent and sincere effort, we move towards wholeness. The measure of our progress is how much we're willing to listen, trust, and make diligent use of our time. To continue to know our self, yet walk fearlessly towards an infinite future.

INNER NATURE

Life is the *eternal dance of consciousness*. Through experience we pave our way to discover consciously our true nature and compile our wholeness. Ascending towards our creative potential demands we continue to explore the *inner nature* of our *true self*. We begin to understand how our minds power can either become a menacing foe that will defy us, or an enlightening partner that will elevate us to great heights. Being whole frees us to bloom like a flower that's grounded to the earth, whilst reaching for the stars.

We express our desires through our body. Our experience of life emanates from the multitude of personality types and behavioral traits contained within us. When we live behind the limited

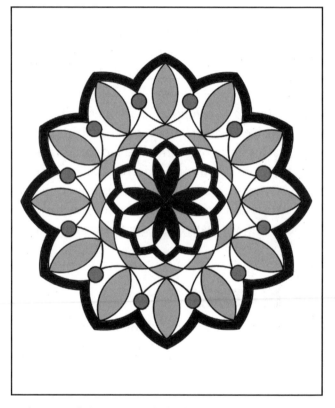

*The mandala is a symbol of the journey of whole-
ness. To discover the true center of flow, which
opens the inlet to experience the infinity that
resides in the heart.*

mask of a persona, the *suit of armor* we wear before the world, we minimize our exposure to emotional trauma and failure. Life however, challenges us to "come out of our shell", so to speak, and bring the full essence of who we are to life. We are dozens of people in one; some we like, some we don't. It is often who we're not being that holds us back and limits us from becoming a more creative person. By consciously accessing our diverse *chameleon nature* we develop a greater capacity to interact with life's infinite experiences. We all have weaknesses of character that at times limit us in life. Our challenge is to live in a way that enhances the strength of our character, so we can participate in life, openly and honestly.

There is no mind-body split. The mind uses the brain to unify and empower the body. The left hemisphere controls the body's right side. It represents our more assertive, scientific, *competitive nature.* The right hemisphere controls the body's left side. It represents our more receptive, artistic, *sensitive nature.* Only through brain and body can we have a truly mindful experience of things, and consciously transcend our limiting behaviors. The Buddha implied some 2500 years ago by lowering his hand to touch the earth that the body expresses how we're relating to the external world and how we're handling our experiences internally. In essence, through consciousness, *we become the body.* How we manage the limitless flow of our two most powerful energies determines who we become.

The only way to know our potential is to *experience all our power.* This requires the courage to live life from the *receptive female nature* of our being that perceives things intuitively and randomly, and from the *assertive male nature* of our being that responds to things in an orderly, rational manner. This is the power of wholeness, the ability to be *firm but not hard* and *soft but not weak* in life. We're able to stay more grounded to the reality of

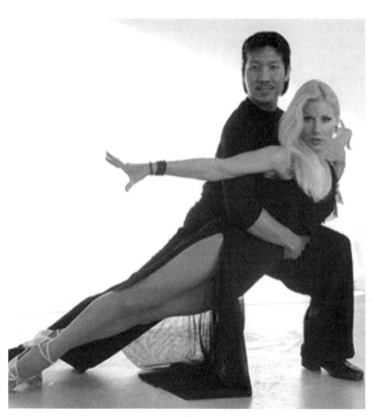

The Rumba is the tale of two lovers embraced in the expression of a desire. Often it's whom we're not being that holds us back from being more authentic.

life with the flexibility to flow with the nature of things. This internal polarity is the wellspring of Fearless Spirit, Joyous Heart. The celestial inner nature to unify, and extend the infinite boundaries of our current self to experience all we are.

To discover the limits of possibility we must *open our mind* to the impossible. The deeper we travel into our inner nature, the more open is our conscious awareness to expand our development. The most important thing in life is our growth. To awaken our inner evolutionary forces that prompt the energetic shifts for change. Each experience brings us closer to a more innate discovery of the work best suited to our nature.

STAY IN THE GAME

There are infinite possibilities in life. By perceiving events and people as manifestations of energy, rather than physical entities, we can *sense life*. We can continue to move beyond our current limitations and stay in the game as life evolves. Chance favors those with the pliable adaptability to change with change and instinctively *step up to the plate* and live life to the max. Develop a *spirit of vitality* with a *presence of heart* to continuously move towards life's more creative realms.

Life is full of phases that require us to embrace change. We need an *alert mind* to capitalize on life's chances and to *sense our response*. Life's critical decisions are often beyond the scope of our intellect. When we think we know something or adhere to set ways, we limit our options. Our intuition however can sense particular needs and create infinite options. It is our capacity to slow down and anticipate the energy of a situation that enables us to sense what's next. Life is the interplay between gathering our energy for movement, and engaging our self into action. To stay

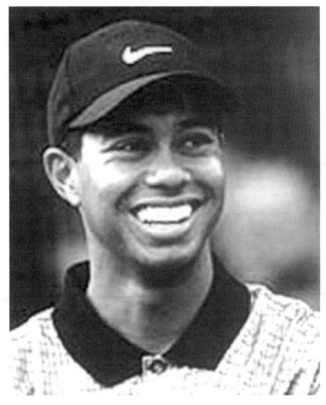

*Tiger Woods shows that the limits in life are what
we settle for. When we aim to be the best we can be,
we improve with time. There are no pre-set limits
to what we can experience.*

in the game and create endless possibilities, we must learn to yield but never surrender. As the saying goes, "Oaks may fall where reeds brave the storm". Remain *open to chance*, and adhere to life's flow.

Energy circulating harmoniously throughout our body has a beneficial effect on our state of mind. The mind may be the initiator of action as it directs our intention, but our *body's energy levels* determine the potency of our efforts. Energy is the prime mover to ride the tides of change and intuitively sense the right course of action. When the body's energy is low, the mind loses the will to take decisive action. As any fighter knows, when the body's energy levels diminish, the head follows. Our *competitive spirit* for life falters. Conditioning is key, when our body's energy is abundant our spirit of vitality rises, with the presence of heart to sense and move towards more creative possibilities, immediately.

To *raise our spirit of vitality* practice the *posture of power*. Suspend the head as if lifted upward by a golden thread, relax the chest and breathe from the belly. This natural state enables the diaphragm muscle to efficiently energize the body whilst keeping the mind calm, yet alert. It also concentrates energy in the lower part of our body keeping our emotions stable and intellect focused. Such poise enables us to stay *centered* and *in-tune* with life's ever-changing circumstances. The right action comes from the right way of being and thinking. Life favors the energetic. Those who gain momentum by picking up their own game to ensure both mind and body are attuned to change.

To *sense with presence of heart* develop the awareness of energy. When we acknowledge all things as being manifestations of energy, we realize that our consciousness forms our actions. In life, *force yields to power*. Refrain from the need to meet force with force, *sense a situation,* and allow our energy to naturally flow. This way there are no limits. It creates the aura of harmony, which others sense as leading the way. It lifts our spirit and strengthens our enthusiasm to commit to life wholeheartedly. Whatever we do in life, we live with forever. Remember, life evolves things, and things evolve life, the rest is up to us. The key is to live without limitation.

LIVE ABUNDANCE

A *river of energy* rages inside of us, seeking the *freedom to flow* in harmony with life. To embrace what life offers us and to follow where our heart guides us. Life is an *energy-flow* of limitless proportions, which we experience as the manifestation of our current state of consciousness. Through integration, we develop an awareness of the vastness of life, with the *consciousness* of *living in abundance.*

Each of us are *born full of potential.* Inside us are more possibilities than we could ever imagine. The instinctive power to evolve is already programmed within us waiting to flow like a river as we come on stream. We are like individual islands, energetically interconnected to a vast *ocean of intelligence.* We plug into this collective mind and become a part of everything, integrated within the web of life by choice. When we separate from this collective power, we diminish our energy and limit the possibility to integrate our experiences. When we *merge with life's greater purpose,* through sharing and caring, we open the inlet to experiencing the full spectrum. Having an *ego with intent for all* is key to journeying beyond oneself, to the realms of abundance.

Our state of consciousness is the abiding reality to manifesting a steady flow of abundance. It links the *"I" "WE"* and *"LIFE".* There are no set-limits to the level of consciousness we

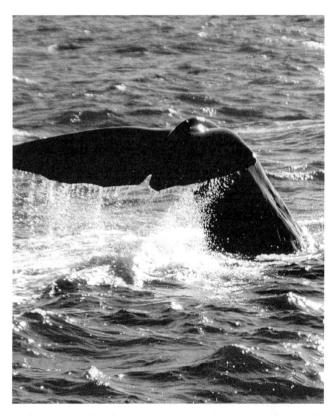

*Life constantly shifts along the continuum, from the
known and visible into the unknown and invisible.
We are our own limits.*

can experience. It can either diminish or expand towards infinity. The choice is ours. Segregation forms a suit of armor, with the illusion of growth. As our level of consciousness diminishes, it dams the river of energy that *our heart knows* should flow freely with life. When we open our heart unconditionally, our level of consciousness elevates to encompass greater levels of awareness. Integration is the bridge to the sweet spot in life, to merge and experience life's abundance. Without assistance there is no growth, we remain incomplete. When we *relinquish the attachment to control things*, less becomes more as life flows freely. The *mind-set* of seeing life as a *continuous expansion* towards infinity is our gateway to living in abundance.

Life constantly shifts along the continuum, from the unknown and invisible into the known and visible. When we live from a perspective of fixed goals and rigid values, we close our self off to chance. It is not always possible to anticipate the opportunities that await us. When we place limits on our self, we inhibit the chance for things to enter into our life. Being set in our ways means we can lack the insight and flexibility to change and adapt with what life deals us. Preconceived ideas about how life should unfold may serve us well as long as everything develops predictably. Life can however throw curve balls that we don't see coming. Energy flows more harmoniously when we *think of life as a flow*, without fixed and definite goals. Trust the process of life and let things happen.

Desire impels us. The key is to *focus our energy in the direction of our intended destination*. Like the surfer who knows each wave is a uniquely dynamic experience, and is always ready to adapt and change. Honing our senses with the desire to fulfill our potential ensures we follow the path of our own journey and live in the flow of life's stream. Our consciousness determines our realized destiny.

SOUL KEYS

*There are no pre-set limits to what we can
experience - open the inlet to infinite
realms through awareness*

*Aligning heart and mind creates the point
of focus that peels away the layers
of illusion and any limiting conceptual
thoughts engineered by our mind*

*The only way to know our potential is
to experience all our power - be firm
but not hard and soft but not weak in life*

*Chance favors those with the pliable adaptability
to change with change and instinctively step
up to the plate and live life to the max*

*Having the ego with intent for all is key to
creating the bridge to journey beyond oneself
into the realms of abundance -
We are our own limits*

PAUSE & REFLECT

What is my attitude?

What do I want from life?

Am I prepared to pay the price?

Who have I become?

How can I improve my life?

CHAPTER 6

MANA IS A WAY OF LIFE

If there be righteousness in the heart there will be beauty in the character.

If there be beauty in the character there will be harmony in the home.

If there be harmony in the home there will be order in the nation.

If there be order in the nation there will be peace in the world

CONFUCIUS

*Being body centered
awakens an intuitive
power within us.
The part of us we call,
soul, that expands our
connection with others,
to engage in life's
potentiality, with
creativity, integrity
and compassion.*

MANA

Mana is a way of living in harmony with the forces of life. It is based upon *self-knowledge* and the awareness of our relationship with all things. People with Mana emanate an aura of *self-ease* that we sense when they walk into a room. Their eyes are soft, and wise, they possess the *honor* and *integrity* able to master the manipulation of their own force.

Mana is *self-power*, with the presence of a deeper knowing. Through the journey of self-awareness we begin to sense an essence within us, that binds us with an even greater power operating in life. This inner essence is often referred to as *our soul*, the part of us that speaks through the deeper wisdom of our consciousness. From here, we integrate the power of our personality into life's grander scheme, with a healthy assertion of who we are and what we stand for in this world. The authentic way of living, with the true desire to *love, understand* and *be compassionate* towards all life. By understanding our self, we can *face our fear* of who we're not, and *embrace all that we are.* Being possessed by fear diminishes our personality. Access to our deeper levels brings meaning and creative expression into our conscious awareness. Our personality is the tip of the iceberg in terms of our potential. Our real power resides deeper.

Life invites us to *know our self* and move towards *infinite power.* Beneath the mask we place before the world, is our original face. To truly know a person, we only have to look beyond their exterior and stare deeply into their eyes. Forget about how big their muscles are, the words they use, or how beautiful they may appear; the truth resides within. At any given time we have the choice to consciously experience the person we have become, to peel away the layers of illusion, and be who we really are. First we have to *let go,* both the need to control external factors, and the fear of wrestling with our self.

Mana is the unification of *head* and *heart*. Our way of living life through our *values* that plot our true potential, whilst honoring the environment and all living things. To acknowledge the pride that defines our unique individuality, and our will to *contribute to the larger whole*. Pride sets our boundaries in life that are compatible with our sense of identity, beliefs that ring true at our deepest level. When we detach from the fear of exposing our vulnerability and limitations to others, we experience an inner peace that makes us more humble and deeply respectful of life. We release the desire to dominate people or to withdraw from life. Our heart becomes free to resonate with our *true purpose*, the baring of our *individual soul*, honestly and openly.

Our journey in life is marked by failure and learning. The lesson is to embrace the truth of who we are. To face the patterns and mistakes we keep repeating and move on. It takes Mana to live and dance with the trials and changes in life, to understand rather than judge. To experience the true power of faith, which is based upon love. Having Mana means honoring life's cycles and rhythms, balancing our feminine and masculine sides. Our personality is created by our mind. The key is remembering our *true nature* has a love for creativity and a relationship with all things.

AUTHENTIC POWER

There comes a time in every person's life when a deep calling signals a need to change. This *time of awakening* occurs when our personality starts to imprison our sense of inner peace, and wellness. It is often experienced as a period of disillusionment, whereby the walls of our persona come tumbling down so a new cycle of growth can emerge. Authentic power is *self-knowledge*,

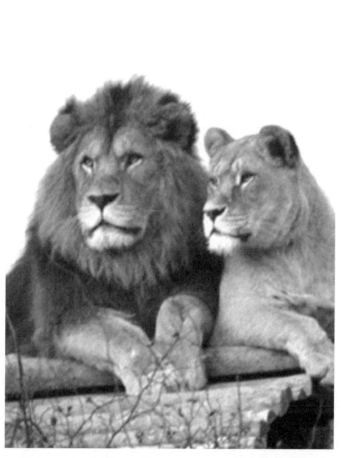

*There is nothing more beautiful than the light of
self-knowledge. Every person knows life demands
noble uplifting principles.*

aligned to living positively, with the full awareness of the significance of life.

Life is change. By *expanding our awareness* and *evolving our consciousness* we can continue to challenge our creative evolution. This awakening process is our window of opportunity to a *life of meaningful expression*. A time to acknowledge that change is an inevitable part of life's unfolding, and that we must be able to detach from things that no longer serve our growth. One of the hardest things to accept is that our personality is only part of who we are. It is our deeper, *soul's essence*, that enlightens and strengthens our personality, to move beyond the realm of "its all about me", into the world of "we are all family". When we choose to live from an integrated state, we subconsciously initiate a *soul-personality alignment*. This way we access knowledge from our deeper levels of consciousness, to bring meaning and pleasure into our life. Our real power is total and complete in itself. True alignment transcends us from being a personality who has a soul, to being a *soul that has a personality*. This way we live deeply and openly.

Mana means listening to what our inner essence is trying to tell us, without needing to satisfy our ego's need to remain center stage. Or as the saying goes, "give our self up to find our self again". By centering our energy, we're able to detach from the idea of being the "center of the universe". Our ego's perspective awakens to a new experience of our self, one that's "centered within the universe". We are all spokes in the wheel of life, vital to its overall balance and flow. Through our awakening, we subconsciously facilitate the awakening of others. We encourage others to *unfold from within* and embrace more.

Life is about taking advantage of prevailing conditions and *moving with the winds of change*. This guidance arises naturally from our soul-infused personality through new ideas and creative visions. It injects fresh energy that moves us towards achieving a higher purpose. We realize that sometimes we act for our own benefit and sometimes we serve as an instrument to benefit others. Every year, each day, and all seasons bring change. Life is full of events that present us with a greater understanding of who we are and our relationship to the world. Mana is the urge to merge and align our life to the path that favors the highest level of our being.

To live authentically is to engage in *creative work* or to *provide a service* with a genuine heartfelt extension towards the needs of others. Any work that stretches who we are, and is aligned towards the benefit of others, brings with it the awareness to living with Mana. Contemplation and meditation are excellent ways to turn inward to gain an insight of the limited focus of self. Authentic power yields awareness for the greater perspective of the continuous act of creation, that's unfolding now.

HONOR THYSELF

Everything we think, speak, and do impacts on who we are, and who we will become. The karma of life means all our actions bring their consequences. As Buddha said, "Effect follows cause as the wheel of the cart follows the foot of the oxen". To understand the truth of a predicament and take appropriate action is living in accordance with *self-honor*. We must *choose carefully* before we act, and make the decisions that nourish the path that supports our highest growth.

Living with honor builds the inner foundation to *live the life our soul speaks*. Being honorable is essential to avoid becoming the victim in life and to stay on course to reclaim our natural state.

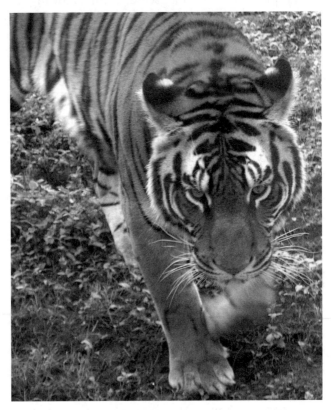

Fearless Spirit - Joyous Heart is the power to face our truths with courage - to face our tigers in life.

Living with self-honor is powerful, because it allows us to question the *beliefs we've learned* with the *truths we discover* through trial and error. Our mind provides the framework for experience, from which we grow. Our evolution is dependent upon our ability to develop our mind and nurture our soul. Self-honor is about *being responsible* for our own thoughts and actions. It means having the courage to positively alter our personality so we look in the mirror and walk down the street knowing we are being honest to our self.

Within us are both *assertive* and *yielding powers*. Each is a part of life's natural cycle of change and renewal. Honoring our predicaments in life simplifies the choice to yield or assert our power. Know *there's a time for everything*. If we need to let something go, then do so. If we must stand our ground, or speak our mind to claim our power then we do so. What matters is *our motive*. Why we do things determines the subsequent consequences. Weighing our intended actions against the possible outcomes helps us choose with moral conscience the appropriate response. As the wheel of life continues to spin relentlessly, we must *face our tigers*, our inner fears, and speak and act upon our deepest truths. Living by right thought, right word and right action, sets in motion constructive and positive cycles of cause and effect. This brings Mana to our name.

Self-honor contains the power to *believe in who we are*. The sacred state of knowing that "*I am*" whatever I give honor and direct my power towards. If we hide from who we are, we will be lost forever. There is honor in believing that life has a meaningful journey awaiting us. The challenge is in accepting that change and the risk of failure are all part of discovering our potential. The important thing is to *keep faith in life*. Faith is the bridge that delivers us the courage to persevere no matter what life throws at us. To honor what it bares and make the most of our opportunities.

The more we *free our self* from the domination of arbitrary ideals and learn the true standards by which we should behave, the more we detach from the ideal state of perfection. Through living an honorable life we find our righteous place in the scheme of things and understand others have their rightful place too. When we honor ourselves we find the power within us to *honor all things for what they are*, without prejudice or the need to manipulate and control. We discover our inner voice that's been there all the time saying to us, "I am free to live this life as me".

CODE OF CONDUCT

We are what we live. Having clear philosophical doctrines in life regarding our *code of conduct* provides us with a strong character base. The moral truths we live by become the principles that form the template for our *way of living*. They serve as the underlying essence for everything we do, as we endeavor to strive towards our goals. Our ability to live a *life of integrity* comes from the truth of our behavior. As Maximus said in the movie Gladiator, "Our actions echo in eternity".

Mana forms our foundation for developing a code of conduct to encompass the ever-changing circumstances of life. It's based on the law of cause and effect, on *being virtuous*, whereby life becomes more meaningful, constructive and peaceful. This means being *warm-hearted*, and morally good with the intent towards manifesting life-enhancing effects. To act upon others as we would have them act unto us. It involves cultivating human affection and respect for all life. Above all it demands the common sense to detach from the need to use violence, with self-defense used as our last option. Mana is the *moral courage* to act with *integrity*, our personal truths every moment.

The *middle way* is the way. As the ancient saying goes, "Too

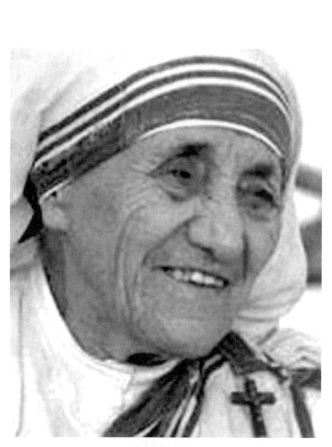

Live the life the soul speaks.
Righteous actions come from the right way of
thinking and the right way of being.

little is the same as too much, balance is the key". The ability in life to know when to be firm in our actions, but not hard, and at times to be soft in our actions, but not weak. To honor where we find our self in life, is to live life with mana. Knowing that every experience has something to teach us. It means giving all we have to offer today. The universe doesn't judge us on who we are, or are not. Divine justice is in accordance with what we do. The key is *self-discipline*, to master our inner conditions that determine the outer effects of our lives.

Mana is *spiritual awareness*. We have *the choice* to live as an extension of our personality, or from the wholeness of our persona and soul. Our ego tends to focus on personal acquisitions, whereas embracing our soul inspires us to honor the impact our actions have on others. When we live for self-satisfaction, we ignore the sacred interconnectedness existing between us all, the mind-set of "all for one, and one for all" felt in our *solar plexus* and *heart*. Our code of conduct determines the life we experience. It is based on what each of us decides our level of consciousness will be. By allowing our actions to reflect a more truthful way of thinking, we awaken our *spiritual eye* and align our self towards creating a future that embraces success and inner peace.

Each day we *face the truth* of our actions. Everything we ever do comes with us at some level to form the person we are today. Our actions either move us towards a life based upon *sharing and caring* for one another, or towards self-centeredness and selfishness. Our outer world mirrors the beliefs of our inner world. The code of conduct we decide upon determines everything we experience. Our way of behaving should add balance to our character and stability to our way of thinking. With life, comes the *responsibility* for all our actions. Live with the desire to assist the growth of others, as well as our self, through alignment of our actions to *principles of wholeness*. The key is to discipline our behavior to conform to our inner self as the mainstay of a way of conduct.

FIRE IN THE BELLY

Mana is the *personal power* to stand firm to our truths. More importantly it is about walking through our fears. We can use our fears as allies, messengers on our journey to learn from. When we divorce our self from the fear of consequences, even that of dying, other people, and situations no longer hold power over us. We begin to unleash the *fire in the belly* that *ignites our heart* to do in life that which resonates soulful integrity.

Nothing meaningful in life is ever accomplished without risking who we are. Our success follows the *sense of purpose* we experience as an inner reality. As our mind becomes more enlightened by the greater perspective of our soul's presence, our personality begins to entertain a grander purpose. The central point from which we *resonate with life* is our heart. From here, we balance the flow of our personality's will and our soul's essence to naturally embrace our oneness. Through integration we ignite the *fire in our belly* to *awaken the love in our heart* and broaden *our minds eye* to life's greater realms. Or as the saying goes follow "the stairway to heaven". The power of our soul demands we risk who we are to live a life of daring purpose.

Fire in the belly is generated by *centering our energy*. The state of being that keeps our *head cool* and our *belly hot*. The way of doing whereby our thoughts, emotions and actions align. What we sense in our core, urging us to pursue what our heart feels and our mind reasons to be us. Gathering our focus unifies our composure and intent, from which resonates the power to act with integrity, now. When the heat comes on in life there exists a brief moment when fear, insecurity, and uncertainty stare us in the eye. Before they can paralyze our instinctive power to act, calm the

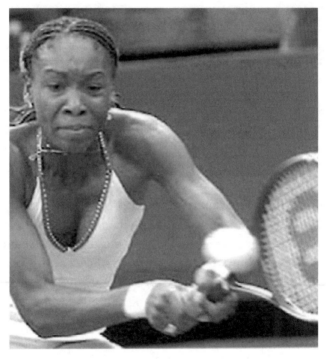

*Venus Williams shows the fire in the belly
that ignites the heart to resonate the
souls sense of purpose.*

mind with a deep breath and make the choice with faith, that within is the power to *conquer the moment with integrity*. Only from a place of integration can mind and body harness the Mana to honor life truly. Keep asking *what resonates* and follow this as strategy.

The *freedom of our individuality* protects the integrity of our soul. Mana is to embrace for our own growth, without the need to control others or resort to violence, whilst endeavoring to harmonize our relationship with others. Life is always asking us to be authentic, to exude more of our self. This means *being sincere* to our self about what we do, rather than realizing someone else's expectations and beliefs. It's about honestly expressing the essence of our soul as we apply our self, totally and completely. Fire in our belly gives us our conscious identity from the masses to be truly authentic and expressive. To live our inner truth as our word and deed walk together.

Mana demands we *remain loyal* towards our growth. The first person we must support is our self. Without personal power we are not much use to others. Having fire in the belly means every cell in our body believes, beats and works as one. It harnesses the *eye of the tiger* that comes from deep within to focus and face anything. To *honestly express our self* at all times. Life often tests our willingness and unceasing courage to cultivate the inner strength to overcome liabilities and obstacles. It is the efforts we make to improve our self through the inlet of personal experience that matters.

SOUL KEYS

Mana is a way of living in harmony with the forces of life - The authentic way of living, with the true desire to love, understand and be compassionate towards all life

Mana means rather than being a personality who has a soul - being a soul that has a personality - It means living deeply and openly

Honor thyself - Face our fears and live the life our soul speaks

Mana is spiritual awareness - the choice to awaken our spiritual eye for our actions to reflect a more truthful way of thinking

Unleash the fire in the belly that ignites our heart to do in life that which resonates soulful integrity

CHAPTER 7

BELIEF GETS US THROUGH

Our deepest fear is not that we are inadequate. Our deepest fear is that we are powerful beyond measure. It is our light, not our darkness that most frightens us.
We ask ourselves, "Who am I to be brilliant, gorgeous, talented and fabulous?"
Actually who are you not to be? You are a child of God. Your playing small doesn't serve the world. There is nothing enlightened about shrinking so that other people won't feel insecure around you. We were born to manifest the glory of God that is within us.
It is not just in some of us, it's in everyone. And as we let our own light shine we unconsciously give people permission to do the same. As we are liberated from our own fear, our presence automatically liberates others.

NELSON MANDELA

THE NATURE OF BELIEF

Our reality is the sum of our beliefs. Our worldly experience and the opinions we hold of people and events, mirror our beliefs. The simple fact is that our mere presence changes our perspective of things. Reality becomes a whole new ball game when we realize we're all participants in this game of life. We are each an inseparable part of the *whole ensemble*. We all look outward from our inner minds eye through the filter of our unique point of view.

Our beliefs form the structure of the life we experience. They either limit our growth or spiral us towards deeper levels of knowing for our highest good. Life, like nature, demands that we re-create our past until our unfinished patterns are consciously solved. This entails *knowing our wholeness*, comprising both our shadow and conscious parts. Those who hold onto dysfunctional beliefs that fail to serve their growth, repeat their lessons until they can integrate their lessons forward. Life is like a big experiment requiring us to travel its process with the choice of what reality we will experience.

There are two great forces at work, commonly referred to as good and evil. Both are extremely powerful in their own cycle of life. We can mentally create or destroy what we want in life through our thoughts. Our thoughts have the power to transform our life. Our most repetitive thoughts construct our registered beliefs, and boomerang back according to the mindful intent they were sent forth. The key is to *be positive*, great people believe in a positive way. The choices we make are based upon our beliefs, which either tear us apart or make us more wholesome as a person. Become conscious of the fact that we have a creative power that rests upon our beliefs. Do everything possible to evolve this power.

The magical power of belief is born from *self-discipline* of mind. It comprises a spirited desire to be a creator of life, rather than a destroyer. Take for example our reaction to someone being successful or outwardly confident in life. Issues arise when we feel insecure around these people. We begin to judge them, rather than celebrate their success. Our being small doesn't serve the world. When we can get over our own vulnerabilities and fears, we liberate our self, and free others to shine. The way we respond and communicate with others, determines the person we become. In essence, we can all become powerful beyond measure, simply by embracing each other. The basic law of creation is built upon belief, the mind-set that aligns our *head and heart* with the *highest realms* of conscious life.

Life requires us to *believe in our self first*. This creates the platform to trust those around us and in the process of life itself. The challenge is to believe that we'll be supported through the trials and tribulations of life and emerge at a higher level. Belief builds the bridge that enables us to grow, to let go when necessary and move forward. The beliefs we harbor within are capable of granting us a phenomenal life. Remember, our body behaves like a magnet; selfish beliefs separate us from life's more creative realms, whereas sharing beliefs manifest heart-felt abundance. The *power to believe is the magic formula*. The challenge is to *evolve consciously* as a person. What is nonsense in the eyes of some is clearly obvious to others. Generally what people can't see they ridicule, because the light comes from too far a distance to consciously make sense of the whole ensemble.

TRUST THE SIGNS

We choose our way in life. Our beliefs set the path we travel and the experiences we'll encounter along the way. There are

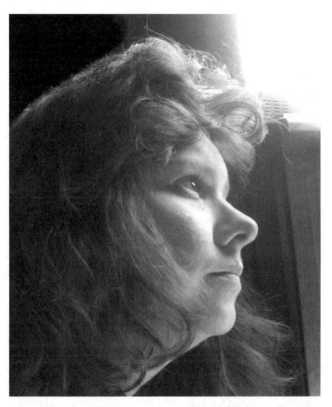

We honor our destiny when we listen to our heart.
By following its dictates we discover our true self.

two roads we can journey, the way of the darkness or the *way of the light*. Fearless Spirit, Joyous Heart is about aligning our self unequivocally with the way of the light, the path of higher consciousness.

We are what we allow our self to be. Whether or not we fulfill our true potential in life depends on the path we choose. The margins for error are small, any deviation in life that takes us astray from the path of love, our true *hearts path*, leads us further into darkness. Into a life of manipulation and lies with the need to control others for our own self-centered needs. The way of light recognizes we all have the potential for greatness. It is our capacity to *trust the signs* and follow the life path set before us, that embraces the highest aesthetics of our soul. The power of not knowing and letting go, anything less is too weak for us to grow. Belief gets us there. It ensures our actions *point true* as an arrow to our highest cause.

Life presents us with opportunities. Whatever lessons required to evolve our self towards wholeness are placed before us. We choose to see them, or ignore them. The signposts to *lessons in growth* come in the form of courses, books, music, meditation, children, our partners, or people we like and dislike, nature, our work place and anywhere we experience relationships. Life lessons are not always pleasurable. They can rock a current belief structure that may have been limiting us in some way. All our experiences come with a higher purpose attached. Trust that life presents us with experiences for the good of our higher development, regardless of what our ego tells us. Through belief, opportunities offer stepping-stones to a life of righteousness and goodness of heart.

Life makes no exceptions. We all experience good times and bad times; this is the cycle of life. It is the beliefs we attach to life's events, which determine the effects they will have upon the growth of our character. More importantly it is our ability to detach from the outcome, and believe that all things that happen to us are for our higher good. As the saying goes, "Good news, bad news, who knows?" When so called bad stuff happens in our life, it may turn out later to be a blessing in disguise. It may be the experience needed to bring *awareness of the truth* of our actions. Not all things that are good for us are pleasant. Life deals us predicaments to reflect our weaknesses, in the hope that we may choose to bring a higher consciousness into our relationships. When we choose to trust the signs, we are rewarded with light at the end of the tunnel - our true self.

Our external life mirrors our inner beliefs. Fortunately we're born with the free will to walk our own path in life, with the choice to release any baggage we deem unfit. The key is to *have faith*. Life favors the bearers of light, those whose actions are based upon love, compassion and understanding. What we choose to believe in gets tested. The trust we place in our beliefs constitutes our faith. Go the distance, face the fear of believing *a higher source guides us*, have faith that we travel the journey that best suits the growth of us all. Deep down we know the right way to live. We feel it in our bones.

CONQUER WEAKNESS

Energy circulating harmoniously throughout our body is beneficial to our mind. It lifts our spirits with an enthusiasm to participate wholeheartedly in life. To coin a phrase, we get to "*stay in the game*". When we rid ourselves of mental and psychological weaknesses we remain steadfast in the truth of our beliefs with the utmost integrity. To honestly be our self, and to live life free as befits the human heart.

Energy provides life support for living the experience of our true potential. We live by our preconceived beliefs and rational theories that we have based on observation and analysis to broaden our knowledge. This is only the tip of the iceberg. The motivational power of human life is submerged beneath our conscious thinking. Within the essence of our *spirit to live* and our *heart to persevere* with what resonates deep inside us, we harness the energetic belief to manifest the latent talents individual to each of us. Life's fortune favors the energetic and those who positively believe in them self. Fearless Spirit, Joyous Heart is an attitude empowering us from the inside, our place of transformational changes where we adhere to our rightful destiny.

Quantum physics states that the elementary particles that make the cells in our body are comprised of vibrating energy. When the body receives a positive input of energy through inspiring beliefs, the vibrations are aligned and amplified. The cellular intelligence of the whole body is unified. The body absorbs and consumes a vitality that develops the minds eagerness to *participate in life* with the *wonderment for everything*, much the same as a child approaches each moment. True enjoyment and pleasure is our natural nature. This stays with us when we stay curious and believe in life. A happy and successful life comes from the rewards of faithful practice and the willingness to *know* and *create our self.* Victory over our self brings joy.

The body rejoices in receiving favorable energy and responds accordingly. We feel open and uplifted. Dance floors, gyms, martial arts and yoga studios are today's temples where people cultivate energy and absorb an abundant flow of life force. Instinctively people know that the body's natural state is to live with an *open heart* and a *receptive spirit*. Ever questioned why we humans have such a fascination and sometimes even an obsession with the *physical body*? It is our *vehicle to enlightenment* of the

wonders of the universe. It's not solely about losing fat and sculpting the body beautiful. Our innate powers run more than skin
deep, they emanate from the belief of the energy that flows from
the essence of our being, our state of consciousness.

Conquering weakness is to strengthen our body's energy
with the *life force* that permeates our every cell. Inner weakness
incites people to fight, to wage war with one another in the need
to feel safe and secure. It's not fear that prompts us to create ene-
mies and perform acts of violence. It's our own inner demons,
and sense of weakness we flee from. Through our belief in a higher way, we realize that *love with peace is the highest energy*. The
only way we can express and experience this is through our body.
We must first *be love*, only then we are destined to live creatively
in peace.

THE POINT OF CHOICE

Our beliefs lead us to a *point of choice*. A place to question
from our heart the life we live. Do the beliefs we choose make our
spirit for life stronger than yesterday? or are they slowly weaken-
ing our capacity to give and receive the joys of life freely? Our
beliefs when aligned towards the advancement of us all can manifest the most positive impact on our life.

We choose our reality of life long before we experience it.
Our beliefs point us in the direction of travel, *life is choice*, what
we experience is what we believe. At any point in time through
conscious choice, we can change our beliefs and therefore change
the direction our life journeys. It is imperative to look to the big
picture and align our beliefs with the direction we wish to travel,
the person we wish to become. In our hearts we know whether
we're walking the way of darkness or the way of light. Our beliefs
either steer us away or towards the direction of authentic power.

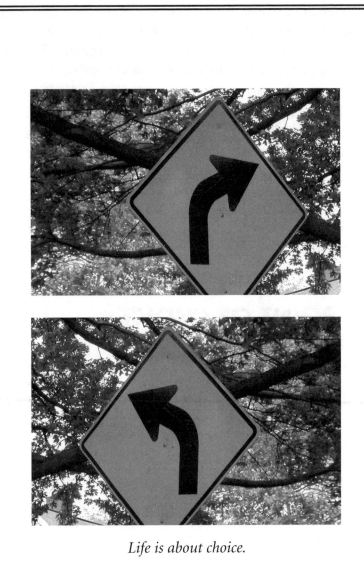

Life is about choice.

Life's laws live within us. To ensure we don't sit on the fence. Life makes us choose through our beliefs the sort of person we become, and therefore the relationships and life we experience. The door to letting our light shine in this world is inside us, contained within our beliefs. Our beliefs set the parameters of our reality. The point of choice is to *face our alter ego* with the realization that we either open the door to the *dark side* or the *light side.* The dark side takes us away from knowing our wholeness, more importantly it takes us away from experiencing the highest universal energy of love. Life is measured by the quality of love we come to know. Only through the way of light can we liberate our self from darkness and open our heart to living a life of higher consciousness.

We are *self-made,* what we believe ourselves capable of becoming. Our journey in life at times can be very difficult. At crucial times we are questioned at our deepest level and presented a series of problems to be solved. We struggle within and around our own talents to gain the ability to grow and express our full potential. When we refocus our weaknesses towards being strengths, our journey of growth begins. To face our demons and transcend the grip they hold over us is to *walk the bridge of faith* and fully embrace with open arms the wholeness of our being. We realize the truth that within resides the ultimate choice, to *solve our problems with solutions* and move towards a future that encompasses our infinite divine power.

Never play it safe, *take the chance on the thing we love.* Have the courage to *live out loud* and shine. Believe "I have something unique to contribute", that "I am a part of life's amazing ensemble". We perform at our best when we contribute our talents towards something we believe in, something that contributes to our growth as well as to the betterment of others. Our journey is not so much about living an extraordinary life; it's about living a soulful life. Our beliefs determine whether we continue to experience sorrow or joy, a life filled with love and light eclipsed by the dark side of our soul. Belief in our self and a life that rewards our efforts accordingly enables us to live life fully.

FAITH FROM THE HEART

The world is not as simple as it looks. To find the way of light we sometimes have to risk the dark. We must have faith and walk the trail of the unknown to our *path of truth*. To honor that life is trying to express something through us that is right for us. Through self-knowledge we can listen to where our *heart guides* us in life.

We can never know the unknown if we cling to the known. Take for example our persona. We can't embrace who we can be, if we live entirely in who we think we are. We fail to see different truths if we live completely with fixed beliefs. What we judge to be good or bad is the same. True faith empowers us to let go of the things in life we cling to and fall into the abyss of the unknown, the void. To *let go* and take the *leap of faith* and *trust life*, the force, the universe, God, Allah, whatever we call it. To have faith that the journey life takes us on is for our highest growth. Walking into this void with faith is to invite the experience towards knowing our wholeness.

None of us are broken. We simply need to *re-awaken our wisdom*. Allow our qualities of heart and spirit to break through our ego's limiting shell, and courageously face our fears. We need to meet our shadow, *embrace our wholeness* and *trust the universal guidance* our heart feels. Living faith is to follow our inner voice without judgment, and to accept that we are the cause and not the effect of our life. To accept the accountability we have in seeing

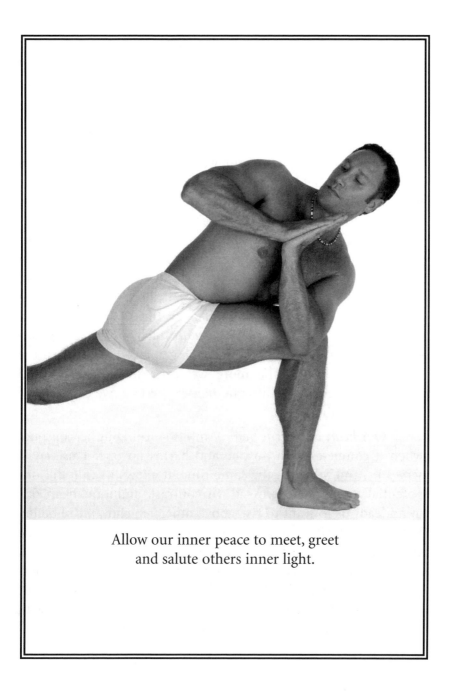

Allow our inner peace to meet, greet
and salute others inner light.

out our future. Faith enables us to face our fears and extinguish our seeds of doubt once and for all. Nothing can stop us when faith lives in our heart. We come to know that the part we've been chosen to play has its place in the scheme of things. We *truly believe* in the process of life and its sense of impeccable timing.

Self-knowledge lights our way. Within our heart resides a *universal truth*, that we're all connected through the center of our being to a collective force, which nourishes us to the extent we honor its presence. Our *soul's power* is the invisible force, radiating through our personality and awakening our mind's eye, like the light on top a miner's helmet guiding us into the darkness of our future. The journey itself presents us with the lessons to find our true path. When we drop our "it's all about me" ego with its self-created illusions of doubt and fear, we align our thoughts and actions towards our *spiritual renaissance*. Living *love* is our greatest *claim to fame*. Like students in the game of life we learn the rules along the way. The more we learn about our self and embrace our lessons in life, the lighter the load we carry as we begin to clear the way.

Our *heart is our true home.* Ambition from our heart is pure when it competes with no one and harms no one. This way it serves us, and others at the same time. It allows us to fulfill our potential to the benefit of all. In contrast, ambition from our mind leads us to want to rise above others, to show we're better. When our efforts go into trying to become better than someone else to satisfy our ego, we disembody from the fullness of our self. In reality, life's riches come in many forms and disguises, richness of the heart rules all. In life we make our own choices and pay our own prices. It's never too late to take another breath, and live with faith, remember our heart seeks wholeness and joy.

SOUL KEYS

*Life requires us to believe in our self first -
The challenge is to evolve consciously
as a soulful person*

*There are two roads we can journey,
the way of the darkness and the way of the light -
Trust the signs a higher source guides us*

*When we rid ourselves of mental and
psychological weakness we remain steadfast
in the truth of our beliefs - to be love with peace -
the highest energy*

*Question from our heart the life we live -
take the chance on the thing we love*

*Have faith and walk the trail of the unknown to
our path of truth - Our heart is our true home*

CHAPTER 8

THE JEWELS
OF JOY

*If we are peaceful, if we are
happy, we can blossom like a
flower and everyone in our
family, our entire society, will
benefit from our peace*

THICH NHAT HANH

THE JEWELS OF JOY

Our journey through life enables us to discover who we aren't, in order to become aware of who we really are. Success or failure, we gain awareness of ourselves through the experience of knowing. We awaken to the realization of our self. We find joy in life when we *open up* and *let our true self breathe*, like the hummingbird who sings a vibration of pure joy as it celebrates life.

Our *heart* is our *center of resonance*. It produces the strongest electrical and magnetic activity of any tissue in our body. Our *heart's joy* emits how we feel about our self, others and what's happening to us in life. Every thought is linked with emotion, that's felt by our heart, registered in our body and expressed through our breath. Physical sensations are the emotions. Everything we do in life either resonates with us or it doesn't. Living from the perspective of *personal integrity* ensures that which brings us joy, is attuned towards the growth of our character embracing life's beauty.

Joy ignites our heart and inspires our spirit. Joy gives us a fresh burst of energy, a contagious zest for life. It creates a *magnetic presence* embodied in our personal relationships and brings out the best in everyone. Our lighter more jovial characteristics shine through with our flamboyant nature free to participate in life. When there is no joy in our day, life becomes a heavy burden placed upon our shoulders. Our heart loses its spontaneity and our soul lay's hidden in a dark cave where we merely exist to survive. We are not truly living. When we "let the air out of the tyres" and *allow our self to just be*, we relax and are able to enjoy things in a more harmonious manner. Only with an *open* and *loving heart* can we taste the nectar and feel the bliss of life's jewels.

Joy is the *unspoken language* acknowledged by our heart. Every cell in our body communicates instantaneously as our heart resonates to the whole of our being the truth of our life. When we drop our judgments of others and choose to see only their good we are rewarded with the paroxysms of joy that reveal the *magic of random living*. The essence of joy is felt in our core, our heart and stomach, and is expressed by the *smile on our face* and the *sparkle in our eyes*. The more we let go, breathe and open up to life, the more we're able to love life and its jewels of joys. Each day practice random acts of kindness, or as the saying goes "fake it until we can make it".

To embrace wholeness, allow joy to be our teacher. Life is a balancing act that requires us to *manage the dynamic interplay* of satisfying our self, others and the process of life, which is bigger than us all. This means knowing when to put others first, or when not to sacrifice our own needs, while simultaneously considering the impact of our actions on the greater cause, that of life itself. When we *learn to dance* with what life brings us, each day begins to take on a new meaning. Life once more becomes filled with the joys that come from living from a place of harmony. Life is sweet when we sincerely know that there is a time and place for everyone to shine, to have their day in the sun.

LET THE PASSION FLOW

Everything we do entwines *thinking, feeling* and *willing* to some degree, as we endeavor to walk the path towards our highest development. When we learn to trust what resonates within, a *creative urge* incites us to boldly *let our passion flow*. Surrendering to the roar of our deepest essence intensifies our courage to participate in life, and navigate our way to living abundant joy.

Our whole being is our vehicle for *self-expression*, the entity from which we experience life. With our head we think, reflect and transform our experiences into sensory perceptions within

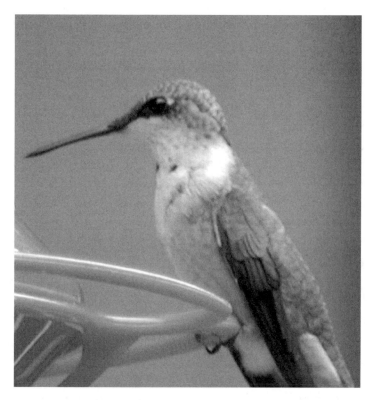

The hummingbird is living example of how to resonate the hearts joy. It knows there are infinite possibilities to experience when one vibrates with the true essence of pure joy.

our core, the *soul of our being*. It is through our core, *with heart and guts* that we resonate with life. Through our limbs, our legs, feet, arms and hands we plug into life and express the will of our spirit. The awakening of self-intelligence to *set our soul on fire* comes through our body. The inspiration to let our passion for life flow starts within as an impulse, which we feel as our inner being resonates a living interest as that moment unfolds. Surrender the need to control, let the creativity unfold.

Passion flows from our core, through our soul's need to *express creatively*. Watching elite martial artists, and athletes in motion, it is evident that to move with such speed, accuracy and grace, creativity unfolds from within, every cell in rhythm with heart-felt determination. We live life through the core of our body. When we center, our passion flows. Our entire body, thinks, feels and wills as one consciousness. When we attempt to manufacture life, we can't, its like trying to light a fire without fuel, we inhibit our flow. Everything we do becomes a half-hearted effort, if that. There is no juice, no soul in what we do. Being passionate demands we *commit our whole being*, have the guts, the fire in our belly, and courageously follow through on our intent. The will to act is the activation of our feelings, through the invisible power of our soul, with every part of us committed to living the event. Feel it, *let go*, and *just do it*.

To experience joy, we must *experience our self*. Fearless Spirit, Joyous Heart is the ability to be fully present and attentive in life with an enlightened mind and an open heart. This means living past the point of judgment purely for our own self-comfort and being able to detach from the outcome. Passion runs freely when our *heart feels love* and our *mind thinks creatively*. When we stop assessing others and experience our self, something magic within us opens up, to trust the totality of all we are that allows us to embrace who we are. Being able to glow with passion demands flexibility of spirit and devotion from the heart. This way our work reflects our love visibly.

We live life through what our body feels and our mind reasons. The brain may be the command center of the nervous system, however it's our *body* that contains the *energy* to feel and do. It is our body that craves to know and feel the joys of life. Passion flows from the depths of our being. Only through the *joy of play*, the physical act of doing something with heart, can we come to know laughter and pleasure. Playing not only boosts our body's immune system, it also brings a sense of self-esteem to our being. When it comes to joy, actions are king. Our body shows the energetic flow of passion that manifests the *magnetic personality* to attract the highest aesthetics in life.

OPEN UP AND SHINE

Freedom of *individual expression* outweighs conformity to any system that molds and limits our personality. The discovery of self through the process of continuous learning and growth is what enlightens our creative mind to transcend beliefs such as "for" or "against", "this" or "that". The aim is to awaken our inner powers of intuition to *honestly express our self* with what feels right in each moment. Understanding our self as one organic whole capable of all things, frees our spirit and opens our heart to shine unconditionally.

Life is an *energy experience*, where we see things from our individual viewpoint. Our constantly changing states of conscious awareness, determines the type of experience we vibrate and attune too. Our challenge is to *look inward* to the dormant parts of us that have become unreceptive to certain aspects of life, causing us to close down and withdraw somewhat. When we address our feelings when they arise, instead of suppressing them we're

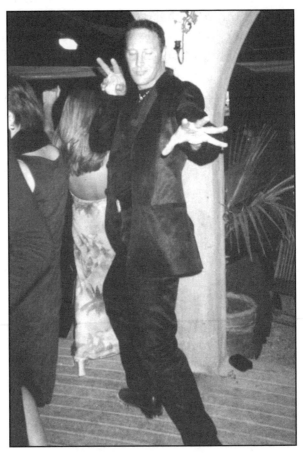

Joy emanates from within. Let the passion flow.

able to energetically *reawaken our self* to participate fully in life. Each of us has the power to know our darkness and bring forth the light within us. We choose our own reality. When we take a chance on each other and share our self, we *feel the joy* that lives between our hearts.

Life is an invitation to know and express our self. Through the inlet of experience each moment becomes the environment for our heart to shine forth. When we move beyond the need to mold with limiting systems that interfere with our ability to discover ourselves freely, we find the sincerity to experience our wholeness. The heart knows that individual freedom means a sense of purpose calls us all. Our task in life is to collectively merge as many fragments as we can encounter along the way. The more soul we bring to life, the more our heart opens. Being our self is a spontaneous event that allows the magic of the moment to flow. Joy shines when we *open our heart* and *share all we are.*

Dancing and singing are perfect examples of how to open up and shine. It means expressing with rhythm and style all that we are. To forget about our inhibitions and let our spirit move freely with what our heart feels. The vibratory rate of music affects our body's energetic state of flow, which alters our frame of mind and behavior. Life is the same; when we open our heart, our mind becomes calmer, which elevates our spirit's sense of inner peace and wholeness towards each other. A closed heart can't reach out, it's only when we open up can we *feel life's energy* from which everything flows.

We can diminish or we can expand who we are in life. The choice is ours. Either we live caged in seclusion and darkness, or we live free like an adventurer, ready for an ever-changing environment. Making no choice is to remain frozen in time, paralyzed. When we're receptive to life, our eyes, hearts and minds open up

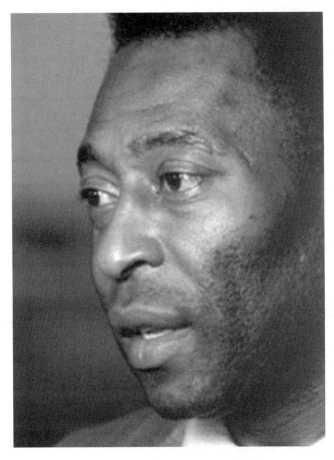

Pele emanates the essence of play

to the joys of life that have been here all the time. All we have do to; is *shine from within*. The study of light affirms the interconnectedness of all things. The paradigm that balances the outside and the inside, what we can and can't see. Both are equally important to our growth and evolution. Our true purpose is what determines all.

LET LOVE BE THE ENERGY

Love is the mystical force in life that summons us to surrender our fears and walk the bridge from the known into the unknown. Into our heart: Our true home. Love is the energy that humbles our mind and opens our heart to know the beauty of living freely with inner peace. All we have to do is *let love be the energy* that guides us to seeing the world through the eyes of joy.

Life is a journey of expansion, a process of becoming more of our self. Loving our self gives us the strength to know there's room to grow. By acknowledging both the things we like and dislike about our self, we bring more of who we are into the world. By facing our fears, we challenge the things that make us feel vulnerable and accelerate our growth towards becoming a more wholesome person. The willingness to embrace our self is the foundation to knowing more about our self. Having the heart to love our self, harnesses the energy to express without inhibition the spirit of our whole being. We experience the *feeling of oneness* as the love pounding from our heart sings forth all we are.

Love is the energy that unlocks our *divine potential*. The internal polarity that governs us like an emotional crossroads is whether we choose to love or hate our way through life. Living from hatred feeds our fears and obstructs love, which compromises our sense of self-esteem, feelings of acceptance and the faith we have in our self and others. Hate manifests as anger, in bitterness, resentment or worst of all unforgiveness. Hate brings suffering. Love brings joy. Our *emotional charge* for things is the switch that fuels our desire to either live in fear or to live in love. The capacity to love and to receive love keeps our emotions healthier and our life in balance. Love is the divine force that clears the way to *become the creator* of our life in the highest sense. Living love is like drawing a circle where there is no limit to what we can be.

Life without a loving spirit is heartless. When our heart is filled with negative emotions it weakens our energy and ultimately our spirit. We become coldhearted and destructive. When our heart is filled with positive emotions it strengthens our energy and our spirit. We become warmhearted and creative. Love is the energy that will *open our heart* and *elevate our spirit* to live happily with peace. Cultivating the willingness to *give and receive love* seals the bond that links us with the unconditional compassion for all creation. When we care for one another and share with one another, we all win. Love is the energy that embraces like an endless thread all life as one.

Love shines light on our darkest parts, replacing the past with trust, peace, and forgiveness, to set ourselves free and *live joyfully in the now*. Love prevents us from jailing our self or tearing our self apart by teaching us to release our pains and liberate our self first. *Unconditional love* allows us to listen with our heart as to what life's calling us to do and be. Unconditional love means that we don't love on the condition that we understand.

This requires *compassion*, to love without judgement and to accept without discrimination. Through love we find the *power to detach* from the known, and instead invite the experience of an uncertain future. Like a lotus blossom that has grown from the mud pond, yet untouched by the mud. From detachment we harness the *power to forgive*, to clear our past and embrace our future with a more creative perception. Love is the force that enables us

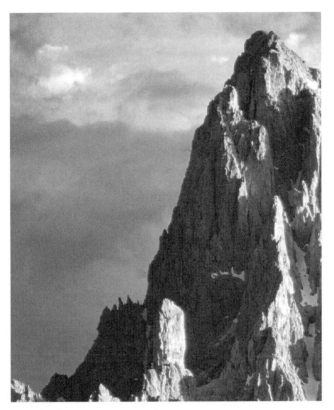

There are many paths to the top of a mountain.
In life there is only one summit - love.
The joy is in getting there.

to experience joy in life. To know joy is to *shine unconditionally*, to express with all our heart the fullness of love. True love is fearless and joyous, *the rainbow warrior*. First, we must be love, for the circle of life dictates that we receive what we give.

LIVE THE JUICE

The *jewels of joy* live in the juice. Look to the realms of art and sport where the more appealing spectacles are usually random and unpredictable in nature. Like the elaborately patterned universe that is neither completely ordered nor has it run itself down to an utterly random state. Life is art that we play like sport through our instincts and intellect. The juice of life resides in our heart, which knows no level or limit. Only what is! – Live the juice.

There is a saying, "the reason angels can fly is that they take themselves lightly". Realize that in the scheme of things we are the equivalent of a speck of stardust in life's ever-changing kaleidoscope. When we "lighten up", so to speak, our ego releases the need to satisfy rigid beliefs. We liberate our fears and open our heart to resonate with soul. We become sensitive enough to *feel the vibrations* of others, and accept people the way they are. By being open and receptive, we come to understand each other, *heart to heart* to live the juice of the experience. To allow what our heart tells us to be truth, realized.

We live life to the best of our ability. Our current beliefs set the limit to the level at which we experience our self, others and life. Beliefs determine the depth, meaning and joy of all our relationships. When we can give up the need to control others and the outcome of events, we allow what wants to happen in life to happen, just because it is. This enables us to *embrace each moment* and *live the juice* of each experience for what it is. The more we push to change our experience the more internally we resist. The

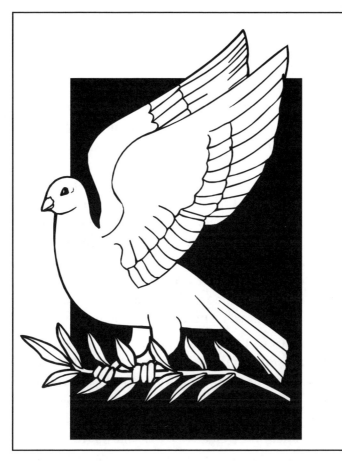

The white dove is the symbol of peace

more we relax and accept what is happening without emotional flavoring and personal agendas the more we come to experience the truth of the situation. We are what we are, and life is what it is at that moment in time. Our capacity to experience what is actually happening is what brings clarity and harmony to the relationship between our self, others and life.

To live the juice is to expose our self to risk. The instinctual part of us when threatened in life either adopts an overly aggressive or an overly passive stance as a form of self-protection. Being at either extreme means playing the role of manipulator or victim. There is no lasting joy in either approach, we lose our power to risk and grow. As the Tai Chi saying states, "The *middle way* is the way". Being able to *act like water*, to flow, bend and blend with what's happening, empowers us with the flexibility to follow what is happening, and choose an authentic response for that moment. To relax, face our fears, and act with honor through the random and unpredictable realms we experience. To risk feeling vulnerable, and welcome life's chaos, whilst knowing in our heart that we are at peace with our self, and the world we live in.

Life invites us to *open our heart* to see the good each of us can be. To transform our life experiences into opportunities and to evolve as a person. To constantly live for the beauty in all things, and see the joy that exits all around us. Everything we do in life, to coin the phrase should "*bring a smile to our dial*". Align with beauty, the function of creativity that allows the child within to live without limitations and worries. To welcome whatever comes our way and dance with the very essence of what it is, just because we can.

SOUL KEYS

We find joy in life when we open up
and let our true self breathe -
Our heart is our center of resonance

Trust what resonates within -
a creative urge incites us to
boldly let our passion flow -
Surrender the need to control
and bring our soul to life

Open up and shine -
Express and share all that we are

Let love be the energy that guides us
to seeing the world through the eyes of joy

The juice of life resides in our heart,
which knows no level or limit. Only what is!

PAUSE & REFLECT

What is life calling me to be?

Do I live my deepest truths?

*Have I come to know love
and compassion?*

What do I want the world to be?

CHAPTER 9

WE ARE FAMILY

6 *Humankind has not woven
the web of life.
We are but one thread within it.
Whatever we do to the web,
we do to ourselves.
All things are bound together.
All things connect.* **9**

CHIEF SEATTLE

HARMONIC ENTRAINMENT

"We are each a mass of vibrating molecules. An energetic body of conscious energy that entrains to biological rhythms, linked within a unified energy field. Through electromagnetic language we transfer information and communicate within the cycles of life's potentiality. In reality, the invisible manifests the visible.

By becoming body centered we harmonize our individual consciousness in communion with the universal consciousness. Like two clocks with pendulums that eventually start to rock together. In essence, the mind is the matrix of all matter.

It is from our heart, the strongest source of electricity in our body, that we tune into this universal energy field. Like Tibetan bells that resonate a life-force throughout our whole being. We liberate our self to experience the divine energy flow that is the circle of life. To be at one, breathe, and be love."

WE ARE FAMILY

We breathe the same air, see the same moon and feel the same sun on our face no matter where we live. Regardless of our skin color, race or religion, we are brothers and sisters living under one common sky. Individually *we are all creators* of life. Together *we are family*, synergistically creating the world we all experience.

Family is the most *sacred entity*. It is the hub of each community, country, and indeed the planet. World balance depends on harmonious family life. When the family is united, the backbone of society is strong. Like the hub of a wheel and its surrounding spokes, balance depends on organization about the center. When we *make family our central focus* we foster the cooperation and care necessary to live together. We learn to trust and believe in our self and others, resonating a warm-hearted attitude towards life. We remove the skepticism and fear that can distance us as a form of protection. Understand that *we all share the responsibility* in the quest to *bring peace to our world*. Each of us contributing to ensure as a species we transcend to the highest evolutionary level of our being. The fundamental principle is that *everything links*. We are many cultures of the same family, which becomes stronger when we are one, and much happier when we have the sense of belonging.

Mass *integration marks the difference* between a society falling apart and a society embracing collectively what can be. As in any family or team, there is strength in numbers provided all members think and behave for the good of the whole. Only through *collective consciousness* do we evolve to our highest human capabilities and contribute to the growth of others. Living from the perspective of self-importance comes at a cost, at the expense of others. Embracing unity means to *look at the big picture*, and be prepared to make the self-sacrifices necessary to

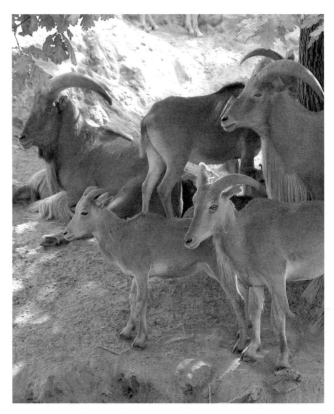

Family is the sacred entity, the hub of each community, country, and indeed the planet.

advance us all. When our actions are for the good of others as well as for the good of our self, we all win. Fearless Spirit, Joyous Heart demonstrates how to live in this world by anchoring new ways of being. We each have the free will to *become the embodiment* of what we want to see in the world. First, individually, we have to become that change, so that then collectively we can then change the world.

Life is about relationships. At the root of all relationships is our intent and behavior towards each other. The key to creating healthy relationships is having an *open heart* with *unconditional love* and *compassion* towards each other. This means to accept others without judgment as to what is right or wrong. None of us really knows why someone lives the way they do. There is a great American Indian saying, "If you want to know a person, walk 1000 miles in their moccasins" only then will we begin to understand them. We must first start with our self, and *make the shift within* if we wish to experience the inner peace and joy that we can then permeate out into the world. We become better people through listening, and our willingness to *do what's good* can tear us apart or unify us. Family is the fabric that weaves and links us together. Through equanimity we can transcend discrimination so that there is no more "us and them". We become the *divine beings* that we truly are.

WE'RE ALL STARS

Science informs us that the composition of the human body is the same as that of the universe. We are but localized bits of ancient chemicals, minerals of stardust formed over billions of years from an ancient evolution. Fundamentally, *we're all stars*, each of us made from the same stuff, only differing in our unique individual characteristics.

The human body, planet earth and the galaxies all exist from the one system of chemistry. All matter is comprised mainly of what scientists call CHON, carbon, hydrogen, oxygen and nitrogen, each in differing ratios. This means *everything is a part of the wholeness of everything.* Human makeup enables us to extract and store energy from sunlight and food, and release it through electron transfer to animate our bodies. We are dependent upon the health of our environment just as much as it's dependent upon our actions. The first step towards creating a harmonious environment that supports the growth and health of all things is to *honor life.* Accept responsibility for our *co-existence with nature,* the state of our water, air, and forests, and make earth a home with a brighter future.

Physicist, David Bohm describes a *holographic universe* encircling both the known and the unknown bound by an encompassing life-force. Like a jigsaw puzzle where each piece has its part to play, without which the potential of the whole cannot be realized. In reality the actions of each of us, synergistically contributes to the growth and well being of us all. Central is our capacity to extend the *spirit of goodwill* towards all people with the willingness to embrace each other through *hearts of friendship.* This attitude cultivates the compassion for all through the realization that *everything influences everything else.* No one is better than anyone else, though it is said "some have moved on further than others" by the will of their actions. Rather than destroying each other through reckless egos, we can encourage each other through goodwill. "An eye for an eye" only blinds us from seeing our true potential and prevents us from living as one.

Each cell in our body is a microcosm of the intelligence of our whole being, a family of cells where each *works for the good of the whole.* Similarly a society retaining a sense of its people, the cells, and its land, the body, becomes a wholesome entity. This

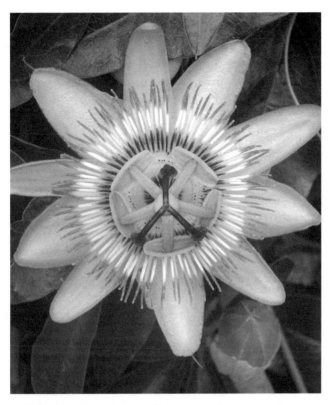

*Nature shows how a flowers seed pattern grows
from the center. Family is the central seed from
which the pattern of growth and integration of our
collective entity depends - All is one.*

requires us to embrace each other and support each other through both good and bad. We are the sum total of our all our efforts, it is our collectiveness that advances us all. We each contain the seeds to happiness, the creative power to live as poets and artists. When *everyone contributes*, the resulting integration allows us to shine together.

We are interconnected to a larger universal whole - *the matrix of life*. Quantum physics calls this the *unbroken wholeness* whereby each part is intimately connected at a deep and fundamental level to the whole. The human mind works like a computer terminal that is plugged into a huge database, that of human consciousness itself. We are each an individual expression, merged within this common consciousness, with access to its infinite realms of possibilities. Through a *quantum leap in consciousness* we open the inlet to experience the experience. Inner awareness affords us the opportunity to know this creative power, and become one with the wheel of life and its ever-changing patterns.

MERGE WITH THE UNIVERSE

We live as a unified entity, comprised of various sub-systems that are interconnected to operate holistically as oneness. We live by the grace of the *interdependent nature of reality* whereby the parts compose the whole and the whole depends upon the existence of parts. Similarly it's the dependence upon the multitude of factors that the universe comes into being. In the cosmic scheme of life all things are *dependent originated*, we exist as a universal family of parts that make us infinitely whole.

Everything we experience arises as a result of the interaction and culmination of *causes and conditions*. All events are caused by earlier events, which in turn are caused by earlier events. Life is a chain of events stretching back into the past, whilst bound to the future. Everything is linked in some way or another and is dependent upon all things at some level. There is no independent, autonomous existence. All things are a part of the wholeness of everything. As Steven Hawkins observes, "the universe has no beginning or end, it seems to fold in on itself". Like a string of beads linked by a continuous thread, whereby a disturbance in one place causes a domino effect elsewhere. To merge with the universe is to acknowledge the interdependence of all things. By bringing our soul to life we embrace with universal intent, the desire to *live undivided* and *love united*.

Life is the chance to *experience the wholeness of everything*. We learn through each other and grow by embracing our individual uniqueness and differences. We become more rounded as an individual and holistic in our view of the world by accepting each other. All life is sacred, integrated into the infinite wholeness of everything. The key ingredient is having *universal compassion*, the unconditional acceptance and love of all things. Living with a genuine empathy, and a sense of our energetic connection to each other, we can accept the responsibility to help each other. We share the same holy human nature as our neighbor with an obligation towards each other. With the attitude that I will help you, you will help the next person, that person will help the next person, and so on until *the circle is complete*. Our love for each other is what binds us, when we know love, we can be at one with the universe. Be love, the invisible manifests the visible.

Oneness is a desire for the *unity of diversities*. Each of us is a microscopic hologram of the macroscopic hologram. We are parts of an ensemble, each of us a self-contained universal entity living within an infinite universal entity. Our actions behave like a pebble dropped into a pond, with multiple ripples expanding outward affecting all they encounter. No one is separate in the universal scheme of things, as *all is one*. Integration transcends all dualism cultivating the absolute non-discriminating one mind. As the ancient Sanskrit states, "we are not the drops, we are the water".

Our future depends on the sense of closeness we all experience. The human body is the field of experience, and love and peace are the glue. Our potential is unlimited, an *infinite experience of possibilities* that requires us to live energetically linked, like an interwoven fabric living in harmony with the unceasing rhythms and cycles of the universe. The direction we evolve as a family is in the hands of all of us.

THE WEB OF LIFE

The chemistry of life, living beings and our rightful place in the universe are still our most fundamental set of questions. In essence, all things are a part of an intricate *ensemble*. The same life, or energy, flows through everything as it threads a single tapestry within *the web of life.*

We are related inextricably to all reality, known and unknowable. Isaac Newton demonstrated how the same force that makes apples fall from trees, also holds the moon and planets in their course, binds the galaxies and pulls stars into black holes. We are part of the same wholeness, an intricate web of life. Science also acknowledges how the wholeness of any matter is expressed in each of its parts, and that *each part connects to the whole through the center of its mass.* Only when we *connect to our inner core*, the center of our being, can we truly connect to others, and experience fully, life's continuous stream of love and creativity. Remember, our true nature is creative love.

We are all *energetically linked.* Each of us at our deepest level contains the whole of humanity incarnated in an individual life.

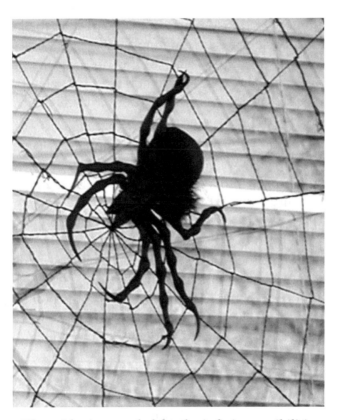

*The spider is a symbol for the infinite possibilities
within life's web of creation. Move beyond
self-made illusions to the life our heart speaks.*

By endeavoring to know our wholeness through self-cultivation, we access more consciously the invisible energy-link that exists amongst as all. The *universal power*, which *merges our hearts* into life's grandest realm: the *cosmic dance of energy*. To dance within the web of life, our body, our heart and our spirit must be totally focused on our path. Nothing less than devotion, total faith and commitment will have us pointing in the right direction. The pathway to a divine future, whereby the world becomes like a single point, where there is nothing that is not a part of it. Everything links in the scheme of things, all part of the circle of life.

The underlying essence is to *expand into this oneness*, and *dance* within the web of life. Like the journey to a mountain's summit, the higher we climb the more comprehensive the view becomes. Each new vantage point yields a better understanding of the interconnectedness of all things. The true meaning of the word universe is "*everything that is*". In essence, everything that is, forms a part of this oneness, with its *benevolent force*, which we call *evolution* behind things. We are but a miniature universe. All that is everywhere is contained within us. Ours is a journey whereby through being human, we've got to the point where we can tell the story. The question is what story do we want to know and be a part of. This is our choice, our chance to dance soulfully.

The whole universe in its essential nature is the movement of energy and information. The cosmic dance of *pure consciousness*, or pure potentiality of which we experience as a manifestation of our *intention* and *desire*. In essence, we are not separate from the body of the universe. We are but a localized disturbance within this matrix. Localised bundles of thought consciousness in a conscious thinking universe. The universe is our extended body, or as the ancient saying goes, "I am that, you are that, all this is that, and that's all there is." Our quest is to *become intimate* with this energy, and to experience this life-flowing essence, chi or prana, with all sentient beings. In the scheme of things, everything correlates and connects with everything else, from which natures intelligence unfolds spontaneously. The key is to let the *heart beat in rhythm* with the universe.

FREE TO BE

Life is the chance to express our *inner divinity* in a finite and unique way. By expanding our awareness, we're able to bring our soul into conscious alignment with our personality. Through *self-mastery* we gain entry into the mystery of this *cosmic dance of energy*, forever free to be the dancer within the web of life.

Integration yields wholeness. Our *heart is our center* for balance, the still center from which we open up to experience our wholeness. By merging our *soul's essence* with our *personality presence*, we crystallize and understand the blessed opportunity before us. When we can master our personality through the integration of our mental, emotional and physical life, and align with the mystery of our soul, our heart resonates to our entire being the truth of who we are. By staying in our heart, we open to the experience that we are not separate. Our mind then becomes enlightened to the mystery, that there are purposes beyond our knowing. Integration completes our oneness, allowing us to let go of trying to control outcomes, to be free, to become the dance.

Fearless Spirit, Joyous Heart is a *stand for the scared*. Everything has soul; all things and people are part of some larger life and meaning. Within this web of life, each of us has our own unique soul calling, which can only manifest creatively when our inner purpose aligns with a global purpose shared by us all. This transformation in consciousness is what calls us all to consider humanitarian issues, with respect to global realities. To harvest for

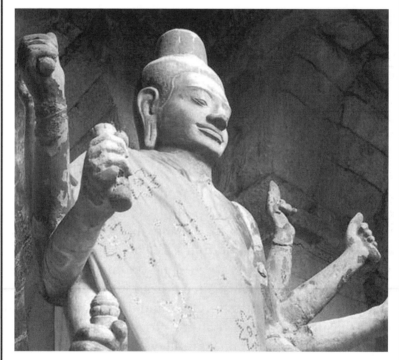

*Life becomes our greatest victory when we summon
the strength to do what we need to do here.*

the collective good, we must express our self as a unique human being for the whole of humanity. To deny our soul's need to participate in life is to sever our deep connection with all things. Is the outer mess we leave for our children, a reflection of the inner mess we can't or won't consciously embrace? The *passage of rights* is our birthright, and it comes with responsibility. The choice is ours?

Time is not the issue. We manifest life. What's inside us drives us, and determines where we go. Our spirit is what animates us, and our heart is what resonates our individual spark in life. By living the sacred way, we can face all our fears, and walk the bridge to a righteous life. We must use our *intellect with love* in our *crusade for life's holy grail* that spirals outward, unfolding ever growing, always returning again to the same point, yet on a slightly higher level. The cosmic dance of life, which contains circles of fire to be crossed, and tombs of old limits to be unearthed and laid out to rest. By cultivating an altruistic mind with compassion, we can change, adapt, and evolve with love.

True peace and happiness reside within us when we *bring heaven to earth*. The key to life's pearly white gates resides in our capacity to *surrender* and *bring our soul to life*. By centering our being, we gather our energy. This builds the physical foundation, which emanates the need to resonate with life from an open heart and creative mind. Only with pure conscious awareness can we enlighten our mind to a more meaningful way to live. The encouragement to continue requires *faith*. It is up to each of us. The key is to let go, engage with *full participation* and *express our self*. Always stay free to be whatever the heart feels, and spirit knows, and we will forever dance with soul.

SOUL KEYS

Individually we are all creators of life -
Together we are family synergistically
creating the world we all experience

We're all stars each of us made from
the same stuff only differing in our
unique individual characteristics

Everything we experience arises as a result
of the interaction and culmination of causes
and conditions - Live undivided and love united

All things are a part of an intricate ensemble -
The same life energy flows through everything as
it threads a single tapestry within the web of life

Stand for the sacred - bring heaven to earth -
bring our soul to life

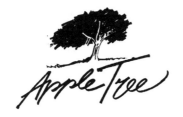

Order books online at:
www.applepublishing.com

"Better Books for Better Health"